I0478646

THE BEAUTY
OF A WOMAN

HER FOUR EMOTIONAL, PHYSICAL & SPIRITUAL PHASES

THE BEAUTY OF A WOMAN

HER FOUR EMOTIONAL, PHYSICAL & SPIRITUAL PHASES

RAY MORGAN OMD., PH.D.

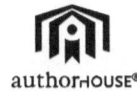
authorHOUSE®

AuthorHouse™ LLC
1663 Liberty Drive
Bloomington, IN 47403
www.authorhouse.com
Phone: 1-800-839-8640

© 2013 by Ray Morgan OMD., Ph.D. All rights reserved.

No part of this book may be reproduced, stored in a retrieval system, or transmitted by any means without the written permission of the author.

Published by AuthorHouse   12/02/2013

ISBN: 978-1-4918-2946-2 (sc)
ISBN: 978-1-4918-2945-5 (hc)
ISBN: 978-1-4918-2944-8 (e)

Library of Congress Control Number: 2013919538

Any people depicted in stock imagery provided by Thinkstock are models, and such images are being used for illustrative purposes only.
Certain stock imagery © Thinkstock.

This book is printed on acid-free paper.

Because of the dynamic nature of the Internet, any web addresses or links contained in this book may have changed since publication and may no longer be valid. The views expressed in this work are solely those of the author and do not necessarily reflect the views of the publisher, and the publisher hereby disclaims any responsibility for them.

Unless otherwise indicated, Scripture quotations are taken from the
Authorized (King James) version of the Holy Bible.
Book cover design by Mr. Reggie Dupree
Copyedited by Ms. Janice I. Dixon
Proofreading by Ms. Felicia Underwood

CONTENTS

**CHAPTER EIGHT: ALONG THE WAY YOU MAY
EXPERIENCE—DEPRESSION ITS CAUSES,
SYMPTOMS, AND TREATMENT**

A Message From My Lawyer

This book is published under the First Amendment of the United States Constitution, which grants the right to discuss openly and freely all matters of public concern; and to express viewpoints no matter how controversial or unaccepted they may be. Medical groups and pharmaceutical companies, however, have finally infiltrated and violated our sacred Constitution. Therefore, we are forced to give you the following WARNINGS:

This book is intended as an educational reference guide only, not a medical or psychological manual. The information given here is designed to help you make informed decisions about your life. It is not intended as a substitute for any treatment that may have been prescribed by your medical professional. The author takes no responsibility for the misinterpretation and deliberate or accidental misuse of the information presented in this book.

Therefore, if you are ill or have been diagnosed with any disease or mental illness, please consult a competent medical doctor before attempting any natural protocol mentioned here. Remember any one of the protocols in this book could potentially be dangerous, even lethal. So if you must proceed, do so with CAUTION and with the knowledge of your doctor.

FOREWORD

Studies in child development outline every nuance of a child's growth and have even given us comforting labels such as the "Terrible Twos" or the "Noisy Nines" as a way of identifying key transitional stages in our children's lives. These studies have been crucial in helping us understand a child's journey from birth to puberty. However, until recently, no guide has existed to help us understand the mysterious process by which we transition from an adolescent woman to an adult woman.

The center of a woman's journey occurs between the years of eighteen and fifty. This is a time of change, growth, and opportunity. As a registered Clinical Social Worker, I have spent most of my career working with women who have had difficulty navigating through the different phases of their life's journey during this time. I have personally likened this stage to the lifecycle of a caterpillar.

The caterpillar has a built-in genetic component that causes it to experience metamorphosis during the various stages of its life cycle. Each stage has a different goal but due to the natural instinct of the caterpillar it is oblivious to these changes. Similarly, a woman goes through periods of transformation where she takes on a different identity at each stage of her life. As she moves from adolescence (bridging the gap between childhood and womanhood) to menopause (the mature stage), she faces the challenges of meeting her emotional, physical, and spiritual needs. She is aware of these needs, but may lack insight into how to successfully cross the bridge during these stages.

Dr. Ray Morgan's widescreen view of a woman's life journey speaks eloquently to all women, as he brings wisdom and a coherent vision of these passages—teens, twenties, thirties, and forties—toward what can potentially be the best years of her life. In this book, he keenly provides a holistic view of the beauty of a woman in each stage of her life cycle. He meticulously identifies the nutrients necessary to properly nourish our bodies in order to obtain complete emotional and spiritual growth during each phase of her life cycle.

I had the distinct pleasure of working with Dr. Morgan, a man of profound intellect, for more than 20 years. He has a thorough understanding of the nature of the female gender. He is a teacher, counselor, and healer and has helped to mend broken lives through his knowledge of the Word of God.

Unlike the caterpillar, we are not oblivious to the emotional, spiritual, and physical changes we face with each phase. We read various materials that explain what we are feeling or facing, but sometimes before we reach or have a clear understanding of a particular phase, our bodies have moved on to a different phase! Because of this, we get lost in a sea of thoughts and emotions. It can be confusing and downright sad that we slide into stage after stage without a strong sense of what is happening. We often conform to how others view us and we tend to wear these descriptions as gloves that cannot be removed. It leaves us filled with frustration, anger, and a range of other emotions because it seems that we are just flowing through life without a purpose.

Go ahead and allow yourself to be immersed in this book, The Beauty of a Woman—Her Four Emotional, Physical & Spiritual Phases. It will unlock the keys to your wholeness and transform you into a beautiful butterfly.

Diana Brathwaite, LCSW/R

PREFACE

As a family therapist for the past thirty years, I have counseled thousands of women from all walks of life, many of whom were confident, loving, and giving of themselves. Some have had a difficult time with life, while others were angry, blaming, confused, dishonest, disillusioned, hurt, and have hurt others. I have found that almost all of their problems were the result of not having the tools needed to navigate their journey from childhood into womanhood and its massive need for a healthy body: emotional, physical, and spiritual.

Often I would ask these women to chronicle their feelings as an initial therapeutic tool. With their permission, I am sharing a few of the notes and letters I have received after my conferences and workshops. Their names have been changed to protect their privacy. These women share their agonies, fears, disgust, wants, disappointments, longings, confusion, love, and faith. I noticed for a time that these women were held in a life of uncertainty, confusion, and clarity all at once. Sometimes their old way still wins, however, for most of the women there are always second chances (glorious second chances!) I have noticed the farther they went along their journey of womanhood and the more they grasped for truth, the more they unfolded.

Here are some excerpts from a few of the notes and letters:

> Hi Dr. Morgan,
> I came to your workshop today hoping to speak to you. I am a forty-two year old woman and my life is a mess. I got married for the fourth time last year. I don't like or love my husband and I doubt if he loves me. We fight every week; he calls me an ugly bitch and a hoe [sic]. He broke my nose last Christmas and

I spent the day in the hospital. He pushed me out of the bed. He hasn't had sex with me in eight months. Dr. Morgan, I wish I was dead. Can you help me? Lots of things happened when I was young. My dad used to hit my mother. He used to call me a stupid bitch. He tried to kiss me once when I was little, and I fought him off; after that he never liked me. When I was twelve my aunt's husband had sex with me. I had to go to the hospital. My aunt told the nurse I was raped by another man. The man went to jail for it. I have a college degree in Social Work. My mother always told me I was too sensitive, and need to toughen up. I cry/laugh all the time; especially if no one is watching. I suffered with depression in my teens and still do; I have had temporary amnesia. I can't get my childhood out of my mind; it was very bad. I can't seem to get that man who went to jail out of my spirit. When I am alone for a long time I think of killing myself. I can't forget some situations and I think a lot about my mother and why she never fought back or defended me from my father. What did I do to deserve this life? . . .

Hope you can help,
Sara

———————————•◦•———————————

Mr. Morgan,
Thanks for coming to my church today. I wish I could talk to you sometimes. You sound expensive. I had a bad childhood from what I can remember, and it's been a journey, but I've come to a very happy middle ground . . . . I am a Christian, praise the Lord, Hallelujah. I trust no one. Just Jesus! I have a sleep disorder, or heavy sleeping. No best friends or friends,

period! I can't be honest about my feelings with anyone and I simply can't find anyone to share them with comfortably. My parents had a drug problem and I had to raise myself and my brother. We didn't have a childhood, I had two children by the time I was fourteen. I spent my childhood fighting off men. I am now fifty; I drink sometimes to take the edge off.

Glory to God,
Brenda

———————————•○•———————————

Written on September 1, 2012

Hi Doc,

Hope you don't mind, but I'm gonna have to do this a little bit at a time, It hurts and it's kind of a long story. By the way, you helped me today to look at myself differently. My mom was in the Army when she got pregnant with me. From what I understand, my dad could have been one of two or three guys. She always acted like she resented me, and I never could live up to her expectations no matter what I did or how hard I tried. I was molested by her brother when I was like eight or nine, and when I told her about it she slapped me and told me to stop lying.

Right after that she sent me to live with my grandmother in the West Indies. It was horrible, what a really messed up place. My grandmother hated me. The couple of times that my mother sent me clothes, my grandmother gave them to my cousins and her friend's little daughter. The teacher was prejudiced against me because I was American. She called me names and made me feel like I was worthless. I remember when I had my first period. I told my grandmother I was bleeding. She said she didn't have a pad and sent me to school without one. I bled all over the place. It was so embarrassing, the teacher called my grandmother to pick me up. When she got to school she gave me a beating in front of the other kids in my class. That night I ran away from my grandmother's house. For the next three days I slept in the park under a bridge. My grandmother's friend took me in for the next month, and they let me call my mother in Brooklyn. I told her I wanted to come home, she said there wasn't nothing she could do about it, so I would have to stay with them for the next six months until she could send for me.

At that time I was twelve, I didn't hear from my mother until I was fourteen and a half. During that time I was raped by no less than fifteen men at the house. My mother came only when I stabbed one of the men trying to rape me; he died and I spent eight years in jail in Jamaica for it. I am out now and live in Brooklyn, New York. In jail, I became invisible the best I could. I didn't really trust anyone. The few times I did, I got beat terribly. This went on for quite a while until my cell mate slapped me around, that is when I snapped (I actually didn't know when it happened). I snatched her up by her hair and beat the hell out of her until she ended up in the corner bloody and unconscious. No one ever bothered me after that.

Today, I am twenty-nine. I have had a hysterectomy, mastectomy and suffer with digestive and psychological problems. Doc, I believe my bad childhood had a lot to do with my problems today. I live in a small room by myself; I don't like being around other people. I would like to go back to work so I hope someone will help me. My mother is my only family here, but we don't talk. I don't think I ever want to talk to her again. I sometimes black out when I get that mad.

Help,
Wendy

Nicole is an eleven-year old girl who lived down the street from my office. She stopped me and inquired whether she could ask me a question. I said, "Yes!" Below is a letter she sent me after our first few encounters.

Dr. Morgan,

Thank you for speaking to my parents for me. They are still mad at me and feel that I am a disappointment to them; I am disappointed in myself, too. They keep saying how much high hopes they had for me and now I threw it all away. They took me to the doctor to get rid of the baby, but it was too late, so they want to send me to my aunt in Ohio until I have the baby. I don't know how all this happened. I am confused. I have been with my boyfriend since the fifth grade but I have known him since third grade. I'm going to cut right through [sic] the chase and say that me and my BF Kevin wanted to know how it feels to have sex. We had sex three times and I got to admit I hated it and we stopped. I didn't know that I could get pregnant so fast. Nobody ever talked to me about sex. I wish my dad or mom had talked to me about sex before I had sex. When I told my boyfriend Kevin, he was shocked and we didn't know what to do. I told my girlfriend I was getting sick. She asked me if I was having sex, I told her "Yes." She told me maybe I was pregnant. She told her mother who was a nurse about me. Her mother did a pregnancy test and said I was pregnant and should tell my mother. I knew I was getting fat, but I was too scared. My mother said to me the other day I was getting too fat, and I have to stop eating so much. But I don't understand, I am only eleven, how can I get pregnant? I only had one period in my life. It is not fair. When you spoke to my dad and mom they were disappointed, mad, angry, and shocked. My mom had a talk with Kevin that was really awkward and uncomfortable for the both of us. We are trying our best to prepare for my baby. I want to keep my baby and not give it away. My mother said I would have to give it away because I can't afford to take care of a baby. Me and Kevin is willing to get jobs, we wouldn't be any problem. I need you to help me again to tell my mother not to send me away and let me keep the baby. My mother doesn't believe I would get a job, she doesn't believe I can take care of the baby, but I can. Would you help me to talk to her again? She would listen to you.

Thanks,
Nicole

Please note: I did speak to both of Nicole's parents. I understood their dilemma, pain, and disappointment. After speaking to them, they decided to let her keep the baby; however, she still had to move out of town until she gave birth. She moved to Ohio and was able to continue going to school. I was able to stay in touch with both Nicole and her parents. Nicole gave birth to a little boy via caesarian section. She returned home and now her parents are raising the little guy as their own son. Nicole relates to her son more as a big sister to a little brother. (She has a brother nine months older than her son). Nicole complains she has little time for anything other than her job, school, and helping with the baby. The baby's father, thirteen-year old Kevin, is not involved in the baby's life. I salute Mr. and Mrs. Francis for their love, togetherness, and understanding of their daughter and family. This dilemma has no doubt created a situation that makes the Francis family stronger. Nicole is now twelve and is doing well.

Where to begin? Dr. Morgan, I have never wanted to be a mother, God knows that. When I got into my late thirties I tried to convince myself that I should have a baby if God would send me the "right" guy to be my husband. This is the thought process that got me into A LOT of trouble. When I first met my husband, he was thirty-one. I was thirty-seven and not interested in having children—well, at the time. As our relationship grew more serious, we decided to get married and the topic of children came up in pre-engagement and pre-marital counseling with you, Dr. Morgan. Dr. Morgan, why did you bring that up? Given a chance for a do-over, I would have been COMPLETELY forthright and honest about NOT having children. Hindsight is 20/20, right?

Four years into our marriage when his friends started having kids, his desire to be a dad and my desire for child freedom both grew stronger and stronger. He is thirty-five, I am forty-one. I felt horrible denying him the opportunity so, I began to pray that God would bring forth a resolution. I even offered to adopt as a way of meeting him in the middle. When he said he was not interested in adoption, I suggested that we get divorced so that he can find someone else to have a biological baby with. He said he was not interested in divorce. So, we sat on it for a while. He contemplated going to see you for counseling (he never did) and then went into fits of anger. He accused me of lying to him and misleading him into marriage. Wow! I was stumped and felt incredibly guilty. I wonder how often this happens to other couples.

I am a firm believer that sometimes God calls us to do things that we don't want to do. This was the "thing" for my life story. So, at forty-one, scared to death, I agreed to get pregnant. After a year of prayer . . . NOTHING HAPPENED!!! Then, my husband went into another angry fit and accused me of not taking care of my body and that's why I couldn't conceive. It didn't help that I am six years his senior, so I really started to believe that. Wow, another blow! I was just a glutton for punishment!

I made an appointment with the OB/GYN and she confirmed that I was okay. She gave me a cup with a paper bag and told me to bring it home to my husband to drop off a specimen. Needless to say, that conversation didn't go over too well. The cup and the bag sat in the drawer for a few months before he finally faced reality and brought it in.

When the results came back, it turned out that he had a birth defect that deemed him sterile. My husband is an only child and this news came as a huge disappointment to his father and mother. My husband is a God-fearing man and he spent some time being angry at God and wondering, *"Why Me?"* While he was doing that, I was secretly celebrating, exhaling, and breathing all kinds of sighs of relief. I felt so incredibly sad for him, yet so elated and happy for me. Our marriage had taken a huge hit, but God remained faithful.

A few months after his test results, he came to me and asked me about the adoption information that I had initially accumulated. WHAT???? Now that he found out he couldn't have kids, he wants to adopt? That was my Plan A and now it's his Plan B? I was again stumped and horrified that he would ask this of me. How much more can a childfree woman take? Well. My plan has always been NO KIDS!!

Well. Again, I felt that God's purpose is much greater than mine. I prayed for patience and agreed to an adoption. We began the long, grueling process. The whole time, I was sinking deeper and deeper into depression. I asked God for strength and patience to get me through this one more time. The first years, I convinced myself that I would be okay if we had been matched. When the second year rolled around, I started to pray that God would take away the adoption and that the agency would find out something horrible about us and take us off the list. I started to dream up ways to botch it up on purpose. Of course, I didn't, but I felt like I was going crazy—that at any moment, they would have to cart me off to the insane asylum in a straight jacket. I had suffered a nervous breakdown in my early twenties and I felt those same feelings inside of me.

Last year, after three years of waiting in line, I sat my husband down and told him that I would not be renewing our adoption papers. Obviously, that meant that I am closing the door. I couldn't keep up the façade anymore. As much as I tried, I had to close this chapter of my life. My patience had worn thin and I was a nervous wreck. He wasn't happy with my decision, but to be honest I didn't care.

I am now forty-four years old and I feel beaten down. Did I make the best decisions to save my marriage? No. Was it worth it? Yes. Do I have any regrets? Yes and No.

Now that my husband is childless and I am finally childfree, we have a whole new set of challenges. He enjoys being with his friends with children, while I can't stand to be around them. Like many of you, I have nothing against children or people who have children, I just don't care to be around them.

Dr. Morgan, you recently asked me to send a note to my pastor at church to let him know about my struggle. I did; he asked me to get involved in the marriage ministry. It's very difficult to be childfree in the church since it's all about family and children. Everywhere we turn, someone is asking us if we have children. And it makes for a very uncomfortable situation when I want to share about my blissfully childfree life while my husband will forever feel a sense of great loss, and is usually offended.

I don't know why God put us together, but I do know that His timing is impeccable. If I was a woman who wanted children and found out that my husband is sterile, I can only imagine the grief. God put us together because He knew that we would be able to weather the storms. We are still very young in our marriage . . . Seven years and already we have made compromises and sacrifices in the name of love.

Had I never agreed to get pregnant, we would not have known about my husband's outcome. Had I pushed for the divorce and he found out later . . . well, all I can say is that I am extremely thankful for God's timing and faithfulness.

We are both still emotionally sensitive about the topic of children these days, but once in a while, we actually laugh about it. He's more apt to joke about the fact that we're single parents and we'll be able to retire early. He is already thinking about future short-term missionary trips and ways that he can give back to society by giving financially and volunteering his time.

I started my sharing by saying that I made a mistake by not loudly proclaiming that I am happily childfree. In my naiveté and ignorance I actually thought I could change my own mind, but as the years went by, the desire for child freedom grew stronger and stronger.

The biggest lesson that I learned is that God has a plan for me. I oftentimes veer off in the opposite direction, but He always makes my path straight. Now when people ask me if I have children I say, "NO . . . THANK GOD!!!" My husband usually gives me a dirty look, but hey . . . . I am happily childfree and living proof of it. The freedom to be able to stay my course comes from the spiritual, emotional, and physical support both my parents give to me. As I look back through my childhood journey, my parents taught me to be independent, strong, loving, decisive, and to have faith that God is always with me.

Thanks for all your help,
Gloria

ACKNOWLEDGMENTS

I would like to express my gratitude to those who have passed along my path through our wellness clinic, counseling, therapy, workshops, coaching, mentoring programs, conferences, seminars, and retreats. Your insight enabled me to gather information to write this book.

I would like to extend a special thanks to those of you who provided support by writing letters, making comments, and purchasing my books, CDs and DVDs.

To my editor, Janice I. Dixon and proofreader, Felicia Underwood, my thanks for your encouragement and selfless hours of working with me on this book; without you this book would never have found its way to the many people who would read it. To my publisher, AuthorHouse™, thanks for all your calls of guidance.

I would like to thank my mother, Dorothy James, Pops William Douglas, my stepmother, LuEster Douglas, and stepdad, Oneal James. Thanks also to my sisters, Angella David, Gail Douglas, Adonis Hazel, and Ruth Hazel-James; my brothers, Dale Douglas and Vernal Douglas; and my cousins, Nellie Christopher-Morgan and Renold Morgan.

To my foster parents, Ormond and Inez Hazell, thanks for providing a home for me when no one else cared enough to give me a place call home. I love you both. Rest in peace.

Above all, I would like to thank my queen, Regina (Ankhesenamen), and the rest of our family: our daughter, Kristal; sons, Nekia and Tobias; my daughters-in-law, Vixen and Hope; my grandsons, Sakai, Kimari, Sanje, and Adonis who supported and encouraged me during this process despite the countless times it took me away from them. It was a long and difficult journey for them. To our oldest son Scott, I love you, I miss you and will always remember you.

I beg forgiveness of all those who have been with me over the course of my journey and whose names I have failed to mention.

INTRODUCTION

This book has been a labor of love. During the many health workshops and counseling sessions I have conducted I was always asked by women, *"Why hasn't my doctor told me the things you shared with me?"* or *"Where have you been all of my life?"*

The human body is a wonderful and remarkable instrument and should be treasured, honored, loved, and treated with respect and with the most natural forms of therapy. It is with this paradigm that I ask God's wisdom to guide us as we journey through the four stages of a woman's life.

Although I am not a woman and have not experienced the things you have, I have counseled and mentored thousands of women over the years. They have confided in me and have shared intimate details about their physical health as well as their many emotions of pain, anger, agony, mistrust, and love. Many of the questions and concerns that these women shared were not addressed before they became adult women.

From the time you are born one noticeable thing happens in your life, it is called **Change!** Your little body is no longer the way it was as an infant; and it will continue to change for the rest of your life. Not only are you changing physically, you are also changing emotionally and spiritually. You may notice pimples, bigger breasts, body hair, and moody moments. Whether you are on the path to puberty or on course toward menopause, it is a road everyone travels. It certainly has its bumps, but it is an amazing journey. Change can be a little overwhelming, but you can feel more in control if you take good care of your body. Knowing what to expect can also help, so keep reading.

Chapter One

STAGE ONE—PUBERTY AND ADOLESCENCE
(AGES 10-21 YEARS)

Puberty—It's More Than a Funny Word

Okay, so it's a funny word . . . but what *is* puberty, anyway? Puberty simply means "to grow up." Puberty is the name for the changes that occur when your body begins to mature and develop into its adult phase. This usually happens between the ages of ten and seventeen. During puberty your body changes, grows rapidly, and does new things. It is very similar to the infancy stage, except that this time you won't have diapers or a rattle and you can dress yourself!

It is good to know about the changes that come along with puberty before they happen, and it's really important to remember that everyone goes through it. No matter where you live, whether you're a guy or a girl, or whether you listen to hip-hop, gospel, country, or jazz you will experience the changes that occur during puberty. One thing all adults have in common is that they made it through puberty.

No two people are exactly alike. The exact age that a child enters puberty depends upon a number of different things, such as genes, nutrition, and gender. During puberty, the endocrine glands produce hormones that cause body changes and the development of secondary sex characteristics. In girls, the ovaries begin to increase production of estrogen and other female hormones. The adrenal glands produce

1

hormones that cause increased armpit sweating, body odor, acne, and armpit and pubic hairs. This process is called *adrenarche*. Breast development is one of the main signs that a girl is entering puberty. She might notice small, tender and sometimes painful lumps or buds just below her nipples. As her breasts continue to grow, she may notice that her waist is getting smaller, while her hips grow wider. Extra fat accumulates on her stomach and bottom as her body starts to take the shape of an adult woman. Her arms, legs, hands, and feet also grow during puberty often making girls feel self-conscious. Sometimes it might seem as though her arms and legs are outgrowing her body, but don't worry it won't be long before the rest of her body catches up.

Menstruation

The first menstrual period, *menarche,* usually follows within a year or two after breast development. Other body changes begin to happen in the body such as clear or whitish vaginal secretions and pubic, armpit, and leg hair growth. A girl may even begin to smell like a boy and may need to use a natural underarm deodorant during this time.

Menstrual cycles, or periods, occur every twenty-eight to thirty-two days. At first the menstrual periods may be irregular. A girl may go two months between periods, or may have two periods in one month. Over time, her periods will become more regular. It may be helpful to keep track of when the period occurs and how long it lasts. This can help predict when the next menstrual period will occur. After menstruation starts, the ovaries begin to produce and release eggs which have been stored in her ovaries since birth. Every month after menstruation starts, an ovary releases an egg called an *ovum.* The egg travels down a tube called the *fallopian tube,* which connects the ovary to the womb. When the egg reaches the womb, the lining of the womb becomes thick with blood and fluid. This happens so that if the egg is fertilized, it can grow and develop in the lining to produce a baby. If the egg does not meet with sperm from a male and is not fertilized, it dissolves. The thickened lining falls off and forms the menstrual blood flow which passes out of the body through the vagina. In between the menstrual periods, there may be a clear or whitish vaginal discharge. This is normal. It is important to note that fertility comes before emotional maturity and pregnancy can occur before an adolescent is prepared for parenthood.

Emotional changes usually begin about the time menstruation begins. During or just before each period, the girl may feel moody or emotional, and her body may get puffy, swollen or bloated. *Pre-Menstrual Syndrome* (PMS) can develop especially as she gets older. Consistently experiencing certain symptoms may be a sign of PMS. Some girls may feel a little crazy just before their period begins. (Don't worry, parents, they are not losing their minds). Many girls (and women) experience a variety of emotional symptoms during their menstrual cycles. Scientists believe the constant fluctuations of hormone levels that occur during the menstrual cycle cause many of the physical and emotional symptoms that occur during this time. A good idea for girls is to make a menstrual cycle calendar to note how they feel on different days during their cycle. Doctors can diagnosis PMS or other menstrual cycle disorders with the aid of such calendar notations. Girls should talk to their doctor if they are uncomfortable or unsure about any of the emotional or physical changes that happen during puberty and adolescent years. A doctor can suggest some natural healing or lifestyle changes, such as diet or exercise, to help reduce symptoms.

Puberty usually ends by the time a girl turns seventeen. Although a girl has reached full physical maturity at this time, her educational, emotional, and spiritual maturity continues to grow. Remember, this is the phase of physical growth and sexual maturation that signals the end of childhood and the advent of adolescence. It is important that parents understand that from birth to ten years of age they are raising a female child who will one day become an adult woman. Since this is the goal, the end result should be kept in mind as they guide their daughter's transition into puberty.

Adolescence—Emerging into Adulthood

Adolescence is defined as the period of time between puberty and 25 years of age. During this stage, girls grow intellectually, emotionally, physically, and spiritually. It is characterized by growth spurts and emotional turmoil caused by a search for personal identity, hormone production, and a desire for greater independence.

This time of psychological maturation, social and mental change, and growth is needed in order for a girl to become "adult-like" in her behavior. The journey toward womanhood has its inception at conception, moves through pregnancy, infancy, and puberty until adolescence is reached. The change you experience in adolescence is extensive and will continue for a lifetime. During adolescence, your body changes are obvious and visible: the onset of the first period, budding of breasts, shaping of hips, legs, and buttocks. As you move toward adulthood, the changes become even more pronounced: pregnancy, midlife crisis, and menopause.

It is usually in the adolescent leg of the journey that things get a bit complicated. Until adolescence is reached, a girl's primary influence is her parents, and there is very little competition. They are emotionally programmed to navigate through adolescence in a prescribed way while preparing for independence as a woman. Some of this emotional programming is positive and some is negative. By the age of five years, she will have received 50% of her emotional programming. By eight years of age, she will have received 80%. By age eighteen, her emotional programming, or rather adult reprogramming of emotions is nearly complete and will have reached 95%.

This emotional programming by parents and those in her inner circle is done unconsciously, but instills certain critical principles that are needed to take an adolescent into adult life. This childhood emotional programming is the process by which a child's thoughts, fundamental understandings, and basic awareness are "soft-wired" into their egoistic minds—soft-wired because through time, it changes, grows, expands, and evolves. Then one day as an adult, she might experience something that causes her to look back into her childhood years and study her emotional programming in hopes of understanding the "error of her ways."

When these childhood emotional programming principles are put into action at adolescence it usually confounds not only the adolescent, but leaves the parents in a quandary, not knowing how to deal with their daughter's sudden sense of independence. They discover she has begun to forge her own reality independent of them. Her parents may be in the dark and not understand why their lovely little daughter no longer comes to them for answers. They believe she is in a state of rebellion and that's exactly what it is. She rebels to wean herself from her mom and dad and to establish her independence.

My favorite psychiatrist and therapist, Milton Erickson, felt that "adolescence was best defined as a time in which the individual struggles to gain acceptance while formulating an independent identity." During the teenage years, a young girl desires a sense of belonging. She needs to feel as though she is part of a group. Yet, she must feel that she is making her own decisions and building her future identity. An adolescent who does not form her own clear identity during this stage may never formulate a sense of true self. She may not understand her role in society. Making future decisions may be far more difficult if she is not sure of who she is or what she wants. She may make decisions that are impulsive or not based on choice. This may result in poor life decisions or regularly changing jobs, marriages, or places of residence.

Here are some important characteristics of puberty and adolescence to remember:

1. **There are biological, psychological, and emotional forces at play.** During the fifth, sixth, and seventh grades, the young female's body begins an all-out biological and psychological eruption in this little person. It frightens all involved—the adolescent, mom, dad and other family members—and may be difficult to accept or understand. Suddenly (and

uncharacteristically) we hear smart answers, witness mood swings, restlessness, secrecy, lying, and changes in their diet, which can include developing an enormous appetite or eating very little. A girl may feel ashamed if she is the only one in her class with (or without) growing breast buds or may feel nervous about being the first or last girl in her group of friends to start menstruation.

During World War II, famed psychologist Erick H. Erickson coined a phase that has stood the test of time—*identity crisis*. He used it to describe the disorientation of shell-shocked soldiers who could not remember their names. Through the years, this phase has become a useful tool to describe the struggle of growing up. The adolescent girl is now between a rock and a hard place with her experiences and sense of identity. It is a major development task in her life. Like the stunned soldier in a state of confusion, sooner or later, she will be hit with a bomb that is more powerful than dynamite—it is called puberty. Somewhere between childhood and maturity her body kicks into overdrive and fuels changes at an alarming rate. With this acceleration of physical and emotional growth, she will become a stranger to herself. Under attack by an arsenal of fiery hormones, the bewildered young girl begins to ask, "Who am I?" While attaining a meaningful answer to this question is a lifelong pursuit, it is a burning challenge to this adolescent. She is beginning to experience feelings that she has never felt before.

2. **It is marked by the appearance of secondary sex characteristics and physiological maturation of sex organs.** It is important to note that the internal and external psychological processes described here happen at the same time her body is changing physically. In a way, a girl's own body betrays her and forces her to join the world of womanhood. After all, the physical passage into womanhood is not a voluntary act, and with it comes new experiences and responses from the outside. For example, before the development of breasts, she might have been welcomed at

neighborhood football games with no sexual overtones. After breast development, the young men see and respond to her differently. The boys may pull her hair, sometimes touch her body parts, and call her names as a primitive mating call. Her body, which has been a place in which she fully lived and roamed freely for twelve years, has now become curved and awkward, and menstruation brings new issues such as cramps and bleeding with which to contend. Most adolescent girls gain approximately thirty-eight pounds. One reason for the awkwardness of adolescence is the fact that this growth spurt proceeds at different rates in different parts of the body. Hands and feet grow faster than arms and legs, which, in turn, lengthen before the torso does, all of which create the impression of awkwardness common to many teenagers. In addition, there can be temporary unevenness of growth on the both sides of her body, and even facial development is disproportionate as nose, lips, and ears grow before the head attains its full adult size. My patients often ask whether they can "speed up" their development. There isn't anything you can do to make your body develop faster. Of course, you should eat a nutritious diet, exercise, and get enough sleep. But special diets, dietary supplements, or creams will not do anything to make normal puberty happen quicker.

3. **There will be an emotional breaking with her past and her childhood to achieve a more sophisticated level of growth.** The life of the adolescent is actually full of questioning the standards set by the parents. Those same rules and principles by which she lived and which she valued for the past twelve years—and which her family valued—are now called into question. Parents must be aware that she is now breaking away from them in an attempt to gain her own independence. At birth, the parent begins the process of nourishing the child so that she will grow healthily emotionally, physically, and spiritually during her developmental phases in preparation for adulthood. Every day, she gets older and moves away from her parents to form her own reality. The parents' task is to instill in their daughter the notion that she is being prepared

7

to function independently in life. Parents must learn to view their daughters as gifts from God, who have been placed in their care for them to raise, train, and nourish providing insights into their own lives.

"Train up a child in the way he should go: and when he is old, he will not depart from it." (Prov. 22:6)

"If you want to know the purpose of a thing, you don't ask the thing, you ask the maker of the thing."—Dr. Myles Monroe

A parent is to train up a child in the bent that God has designed for that child. In other words, parents should rear their daughters by studying and nurturing the unique gifts and abilities inherent in her. Remember, a child is not here to live out her parents' fantasies and end up losing theirs in the end. A girl's parents may want her to be a doctor, but she may be wired to be an artist. So parents must observe closely and pay attention to her talents and needs in order to train her in her own framework. Encourage, foster, and bring out the best in her. God has given parents the ability to be the caretaker so it is up to you to produce the very best individual you can by studying the character and personality of your daughter. See and train your daughter not as she is, but rather as what she can become. This will enable your daughter to become a productive and strong adult woman.

God has taken the time to create each child for a purpose and that is why He has hand-picked each parent. Children are very special since they are a gift of God. (Psalm127:3). God is involved in every person's life from the beginning, and this makes everyone very special from the beginning. In adolescence, a girl begins to question her parent's standards. This is necessary in order for them to attain their independence. Remember now, if she did everything her parents said, she would be a clone of them and act as their little robot, enmeshed into their lives not knowing where their life ends and hers begins.

Her independence means questioning their principles; sifting them through some of her peer group principles and coming out with what she think is good for her. She will try some things and fail at some of them, realizing that some of the things they said were right. Then she will take them and embrace them because it will be from her own experience. She has to be given room to do this, even if she sometimes reinvents the wheel.

Is it any wonder millions of mothers and fathers fear their daughter's adolescent years? Like these parents, you may be wondering how your relationship suddenly became so complicated. "In the blink of an eye, everything changed between the two of you," says Roni Cohen-Sandler, Ph.D. "Out went the easy chats, holding hands on walks, and keeping her secrets. In came slammed doors, exasperated sighs, sullen moods, and rude comments. These changes are mystifying and devastating to parents."

What does a parent do when their teenage daughter is spinning out of control, and nothing is bringing her back? Some girls transform from a sweet, ribbon-wearing, kiss-giving, doll-loving little girl to a young woman who is angry, secretive, or untrustworthy. Parents handle this predicament in many ways as their adolescent daughter seeks out and implements her own independence. Some understand that adolescence is a time of using discord as a means of testing the relational waters between you and her. Girls will often put out information designed to irritate one or both parents. Whether she does this consciously or unconsciously, her goal is to see if you can be trusted with what is on her mind. If you overreact, then you may lose her trust. Deciphering her hidden messages requires you to be both sensitive and empathic when she goes into her adolescent moods. Remaining calm and having self-control is the most effective way to help her to open up and share her heart with you.

Let's Look at Her Behavior

As parents, you may shake your heads because you cannot figure out why your precious little girl is acting in such an unreasonable way, or why some students indulge in risky behavior at school. This is because there is a role reversal between the frontal lobe and the amygdala in the brain. Because of this role reversal, the adolescent may misinterpret things that parents or educators say, or the way they look.

Let's Look at Her Brain

Researcher Robert Ruder found by showing adolescents pictures of faces with different emotional expressions (such as, anger, sadness, surprise, fear, etc.) that adolescents mistook "fear" and "surprise" as "anger". For example, as a parent you might say, "Wow!" with a surprised look. This in turn may be interpreted by your daughter as an angry disapproval of her. You might then receive a defensive response in return from her: "I don't care what you think,"—followed by a bedroom door slamming. With that response you might ask, "What did I say?" Think of her teacher for a moment, her teacher's inquisitive look might be interpreted as the teacher being angry. Your daughter might then react by refusing to finish the lesson because "my teacher doesn't like me." These examples also demonstrate that the transition the child is going through can be just as taxing on the parent and teacher. The once tender and loving middle-school student can become quite a different person.

The misinterpretation of verbal and facial expressions results from adolescents processing emotions in a different part of the brain than adults. As adults, we use the rational part of the brain called the *frontal lobe*. The adolescents use the part that deals with fear and anger, the *amygdala*. As stated above, this is generally known as the place where we experience "flight or fight." The frontal lobe of young adolescents is being reorganized as they go through puberty; the amygdala is taking the place of the frontal lobe. Development of the self-system (self-concept, self-esteem, and identity) takes center stage during this time.

When these signs begin to appear, it may not look like it, but the adolescent child is showing her first signs of maturity, and therefore needs patience and guidance even when she rejects her parent. She has to be able to know what she feels instead of what she is supposed to feel, and think what she thinks instead of what she is supposed to think. That means she has to resist what her parents say to some extent. Though it comes in an angry way, she is actually casting off the past and the things she has learned for a while. She is casting them off to be able to discover adulthood for herself, and believe me it's okay, because you are there to guide her through this phase. She will experiment with some things of which you know nothing. Most parents are insulated from the things their children are doing and are not aware of the risky things their children are involved in until the child tells them. Always remember, God is working, protecting, and watching when and where you cannot.

Your daughter is asking the right question: "Who am I?" She wants to know how she fits in at home, in the classroom and in the world. She is trying to understand what is unique about her while at the same time wanting to be like everyone else.

She might go about this by trying on different hats, trying for the perfect fit, the perfect laugh, walk, and talk. She tries out wearing distinctive clothing that may look odd. Sometimes becoming herself takes coloring her hair, body piercings, and tattoos. This process of forming an identity also takes into account how well she does in school, how well she is accepted by you, her peers, and the negative or positive feedback she receives from adults. Remember, as she goes through her adolescent years, the amygdala and the frontal lobe will reorganize as she goes from concrete to abstract thinking.

Why This Phase is Especially Hard for Both Mother and Daughter

According to Dr. Sandler, there are several reasons why daughters and mothers develop conflict during adolescence. The most common are: **You think she hates you.** Dads are somewhat exempt from the emotional roller coaster of adolescence. Mom, the emotional caretaker of the family, typically sits at the helm throughout the adolescent process, anxiously steering the family's course through the maelstrom of the adolescent years. As such, she often takes the responsibility for ensuring that each member survives and even thrives during growing years. Consequently, mothers often feel a dramatically increased burden during their daughters' adolescence.

Her development affects you. It is no easy road to live with and give direction to an individual who is undergoing rapid changes in how she looks, thinks, and feels. On the most obvious level, a girl's maturing body, vitality, and burgeoning sexuality tend to make mom uncomfortable. Just when girls are blossoming into shapely young women, mothers are often in or approaching mid-life. It may be difficult to live with adolescent daughters who remind them of their ever-diminishing youth.

You think it's personal. Mothers typically describe feeling scrutinized by their teens. My sister once stated, "My daughter thinks she is a microscope and I am her specimen; she points out every flaw in my life when we are together." A daughter's effort to develop her own individuality motivates her to examine her mother's every action. This is a far cry from her early childhood, when mom frequently could do no wrong or was the "best mother in the world." As an adolescent she calls her the "worst mother in the world."

Conflict is always hard. In general, it is always difficult time for a mother when handling conflict and anger between her daughter and herself; therefore, they regard their teenage daughter's challenging behavior or outright hostility as particularly unwelcome. Thinking back to when her daughter was a little girl, she expected her to get into squabbles with her peers and siblings. Now that she has reached adolescence, she may be expected to be beyond all that. She should know how to get along with people, especially her mother. This reminds me of an excerpt from one of my favorite books, "Hurt People Hurt People" by Sandra Wilson, Ph.D.

> *"I have always viewed my daughter in a positive light as she moves into and through all stages," says Brenda Hall, a mother from Brooklyn, NY. However, this is the most challenging phase thus far. At sixteen my daughter has an adult body but she is still in many ways a child. We have had some tough situations. When*

things get out of hand, I simply lay down the law and remind her who the parent is. Fortunately, these times are few and far between because of the mutual respect we have for each other. In a nutshell, the key to getting through these tough times is trust and communication. If you can do this, I believe you [both] will 'survive' and most importantly grow in the process."

A Conversation with Your Daughter about Puberty

It seems like just yesterday you were reading to your little girl *Goin' Someplace Special* by Patricia C. McKissack or *Something Beautiful* by Sharon Dennis Wyeth. Now right before your very eyes she is growing into a woman. As she develops, your daughter is bound to have questions about her physical and emotional changes during puberty. As a parent, it is your job to listen to her concerns and keep the lines of communication open. Here are some tips on how to make that happen:

Answer questions openly and honestly. Let your daughter know that you are available at any time to talk, but also schedule time to talk. (Don't always wait for her to initiate the discussion). If she has questions or concerns that you can't answer, let her know you don't know at this time but you will find out. Talking with her doctor may help provide reassurance, but always get back to her with answers.

If you haven't already, start the talk early. By the time a girl is eight years old, she should know what bodily changes are associated with puberty. That may seem young, but some early bloomers are already wearing training bras at that age. As a conversation starter, you might tell your daughter what puberty was like for you when you were growing up.

Talk about menstruation before she gets her period. Girls who are unaware of their impending period can be frightened by the sight and location of blood. Most girls get their first period when they are twelve or thirteen years old; others get it as early as age nine or as late as age sixteen.

Make it practical. Most girls are interested in practical matters, like how to find a bra that fits and what to do if they get their first period at school. Your daughter will appreciate concrete assistance, such as taking a measurement for a bra or getting some pads that she can stash in her backpack or locker, just in case.

Offer reassurance. Girls often express insecurity about their appearance as they go through puberty. Some develop breasts at a younger age or get their period early, while others may not start until they are a little older. Assure your daughter that there is a huge amount of variation in the timing of these milestones. Everyone goes through them, but not always at the same pace.

If you are not entirely comfortable having a conversation about puberty, practice what you want to say first or ask your doctor for advice. Remember, it is important to talk about puberty—and the feelings associated with it—as openly as possible so that your daughter will be prepared for the changes ahead.

Be the Grown-Up and Stay Connected

Even when it feels like it, all is not lost. With a bit of understanding, loving gestures, and compromise you can be a part of your daughter's world.

According to Naomi Drew, author of *Hope and Healing: Peaceful Parenting in an Uncertain World*, the most critical key of all is to find ways to enter your child's world. "Listen to her music with her, even if you hate it," says Drew. "Do some activities together that she likes, even if they're things you don't normally do like window shopping at the mall. Take a genuine interest in what movies motivate her interest. Each time you step into her world you create increased trust and openness, even if you can't see it right away."

Chapter Two

THE FEMALE SEX ORGANS

Has this ever happened to you? You are dressing for a date, you pull on your favorite jeans and can no longer button them. Perhaps you are running down the soccer field when you notice that your legs rub together in a way they never did before. Maybe when you look in the mirror it seems as though your pores are taking over your face. If you've ever felt out of step with your body, you're not alone.

Growing Up and Out (or Not)

Most adolescents are prepared to deal with the obvious physical changes of growing up. Girls expect their breasts to grow and guys expect to become more muscular. But the body often goes through *other* changes before, during, and after puberty than the obvious physical changes of growing up. They may notice themselves growing in unfamiliar places, such as the butt or belly. Or they may grow taller and thinner. Some adolescents get a temporary layer of fat to prepare the body for a growth spurt. Most girls fill out permanently and even if they eat healthy foods and work out, they still gain weight. Still others chow down on everything in sight and remain slim. Eventually it all balances out and most adolescent girls adjust to how their new body moves and works, but it can take some getting used to. What happens to adolescents physically during puberty can influence how a girl feels about her body and herself for a long time to come.

Case in Point

Take Crystal, for example. She was an accomplished dancer with her heart set on following her mother's career as a ballerina. At thirteen, however, Crystal grew several inches taller and developed the kind of figure most girls long for, unless they're dancers. Crystal's friends envied her curves, but Crystal felt heavy and awkward. Now sixteen, Crystal says it took her longer to get over the false perception of herself as a fat, tall girl than it did to let go of her dreams of being a dancer.

Female Breast Development Stages

Puberty always brings many surprises in a girl's life and breast development is one of them. Breast development in a girl is a physical change in her body that starts even before the menstruation cycle. The function of a woman's breasts is to produce milk for breastfeeding. There are different stages of breast development but the development may differ in every single girl. Some girls may develop earlier than others as it also depends upon the overall growth and development of the body. Girls undergoing this transformation may feel scared and embarrassed because they do not know how to deal with this situation. Hence, it is the responsibility of her mom or another adult female member of her family to help her understand what is happening with her body.

There are different stages of breast development in girls that are a part of the whole process of puberty. Some girls may find it painful and scary, but this is a normal process that every girl has to go through. Breast development in girls is divided into five stages.

Stage One

Girls under ten years of age fall into this category. This stage is considered the preadolescent stage of a girl. There is no growth of breasts at this stage. The nipples are little brown buds that are not so prominent. Some girls may observe some growth due to the early onset of puberty, however this growth is unusual. Girls who feel some changes in their breasts need not worry as this is normal at this stage.

Stage Two
Girls from eight to thirteen years are in the second stage of breast development. This is a stage when a girl enters the puberty age. Her breasts are enlarging with buds appearing, nipples are raised and the *areola,* the dark part that surrounds the nipples, becomes enlarged. In this stage, the tissues start developing and are prominently seen. This growth can be accompanied with breast pain. The milk duct also develops at this stage. Some girls' breasts may develop more than normal due to obesity, which causes the early secretion of puberty hormones.

Stage Three
Girls from twelve to fourteen years of age fall into this category. This is the adolescent stage of a child. A girl usually enters the menstruation period in this stage. Her breasts are seen growing and are more visible. The areola spreads more and the breasts start bulging out, but still the shape of the breast is not achieved. The glandular tissues rise up and the estrogen hormone starts giving sculpture to the breast. This can be a painful stage for some girls as they may feel pain all the time.

Stage Four
Girls from twelve to fifteen years of age are in the fourth stage of breast development. The breast keeps on growing and a second layer or mound is observed over the breast. There may be considerable breast pain as the skin stretches and the breast enlarges. This may also result in stretch marks which will diminish with time. It is the *adipose tissue* that gives the breast its dome-like structure. At this stage, the girl should start wearing a bra to prevent breast injury. A bra supports the breast and also gives it its proper shape.

There are several factors that determine the size of the breast, whether it is an A, B, C, or D cup. You can consult a professional for help in sizing and fitting. A mother or other female adult should be very involved in her girl's life at this stage and should take this opportunity to talk to her about every aspect of puberty. She should explain and show her how to perform a self-examination of her breasts. Girls who have not started their menstruation cycle will probably start their cycle in this stage. At age ten, girls should learn how to handle and take care of their bodies.

Stage Five
Girls from fourteen to eighteen years of age fall into this category. At this stage her breasts should be matured, although in some girls, complete growth of breasts will take place in the early twenties. The breast is now round in shape with raised nipples. At this stage, these women will be able to determine their actual breast size. The growth of the breast totally depends on the weight gain and the weight loss of the woman, which means that fat disposition, plays an important role in the formation of bigger breasts after this stage. The breast will not fully develop until or during pregnancy. This last stage may consist of small lump formations, which are the result of complete development of the duct which takes place at the time of pregnancy.

It is unusual to see women forty-five and older with breasts that are erect. The truth is that after age thirty-five, which is the midpoint of life for the average woman, the estrogen level begins to drop gradually. As the estrogen level drops, so goes the dome-like structure of the breast, along with the hormone balance of the body. She can test her hormone balance by doing the weight loss diet she did at age twenty. She will find that she will not lose the weight as easily she did in her twenties and will have to cut back on the type of food she eats by counting calories.

In my opinion, women should begin to make changes in their diets around the age of thirty. I recommend a diet free of mucous, with plenty of fruits, vegetables, grains nuts, and seeds. I have noticed that girls raised on these types of foods do not suffer from acne or other skin problems, cramps, or other systemic misery during their teen years. They also tend to exhibit less anger and mood swings. I would also recommend drinking a daily cup or more of red raspberry leaf tea and blessed thistle tea. These teas supply the estrogen materials her body will require. The taste of the teas are very pleasant. They can be sweetened, cooled with ice, and are a healthy substitute for soft drinks. For girls that crave chocolate; licorice root is a much better snack and tastes just as good. It also helps to relieve nervous tension. Other helpful herbs during adolescence that will give her changing body the needed hormones and relieve tension and cramps during her menstrual cycle are black cohosh, chaparral, cramp bark, squaw vine, true unicorn, valerian, and wild yam. I would also recommend adding approximately 400 mg of flax seed oil daily. Don't forget to visit the office of a qualified naturopath or homeopath to work on nutritional needs and correct balance zones and meridians in the body.

Pregnancy and Breast Development

During the menstruation cycle the breast becomes lumpy, and some may even feel a change in the breast texture. This is very normal as the breast tries to prepare for pregnancy. If pregnancy does not occur, the breast returns to normal size. The breast is not yet fully developed even after completing all the five stages of puberty and reaching adulthood. Complete development of breasts takes place during pregnancy. Due to the hormone progesterone, breasts undergo many changes during pregnancy and achieve maturation. The breast starts swelling due to the development of milk ducts. One can also find swelling, enlargement and darkening of the areola. All these changes help the breast to get fully prepared for producing milk for the baby.

Each girl's body may follow a different pattern of breast development, therefore you may find the ages in all of the stages overlapping. After the age of forty, the breast size starts decreasing as the milk duct starts drying. Later, in the older stage, the breast will become loose and will drop down due to the effect of gravity. If you want to retain your breast size the same as it was at eighteen years of age, then try some breast firming exercises. While exercises can be very effective, don't expect them to be what they were at age eighteen.

The Female Reproductive System

It is important to understand that all living things reproduce. Reproduction is a process by which organisms make more organisms like themselves. The process of reproduction is one of the things that set living things apart from non-living matter. But even though the reproductive system is essential to keeping a species alive, unlike other body systems, it is not essential to keeping an individual alive.

In the human reproductive process, two kinds of sex cells, or *gametes*, are involved. The male gamete, or sperm, and the female gamete, the egg or *ovum*, meet in the female's reproductive system to create a new individual. Both the male and female reproductive systems are essential for reproduction. The female needs a male to fertilize her egg, even though it is she who carries the offspring through pregnancy and childbirth. Human beings like other organisms, pass certain characteristics of themselves to their children through their genes. The genes that parents pass along are what make their children similar to others in their family. This is called *DNA*. They also are what make each child unique. These genes come from the male's sperm and the female's egg. Most species have two sexes: male and female. Each sex has its own unique reproductive system. They are different in shape and structure, but both are specifically designed to produce, nourish, and transport either the egg or sperm.

Components of the Female Reproductive System

Unlike the male, the female reproductive system is located entirely in the pelvis. The *external* part of the female reproductive organs is called the *vulva*, which means "covering." Located between the legs, the vulva covers the opening to the vagina and other reproductive organs located inside her body. The fleshy area located just above the top of the vaginal opening is called the *mons pubis*. Two pairs of skin flaps called the *labia* (which means lips) surround the vaginal opening. The *clitoris*, a small sensory organ, is located toward the front of the vulva where the folds of the labia join. Between the labia are openings to the urethra (the canal that carries urine from the bladder to the outside of the body) and vagina. Once girls become sexually mature, the outer labia and the mons pubis are covered by pubic hair. The female's *internal* reproductive organs are the vagina, uterus, fallopian tubes, and ovaries.

The *vagina* is a muscular, hollow tube that extends from the vaginal opening to the uterus. The vagina is about three to five inches (eight to twelve centimeters) long in a grown woman. It has muscular walls enabling it to expand and contract. This ability to become wider or narrower allows the vagina to accommodate something as slim as a tampon and as wide as a baby. The vagina's muscular walls are lined with mucous membranes, which keep it protected and moist.

The Vagina Serves Three Purposes

The vagina's three purposes are: 1) It is where the penis is inserted during sexual intercourse; 2) It is the pathway that a baby takes out of a woman's body during childbirth, called the birth canal, and; 3) It provides the route for the menstrual blood (the period) to flow or to leave the body from the uterus.

A thin sheet of tissue with one or more holes in it, called the *hymen*, partially covers the opening of the vagina. Hymens are often differ from female to female. Most women find their hymens have stretched or torn after their first sexual experience. A torn or stretched hymen may bleed a little. This usually causes little, if any, pain. Some women who have had sexual intercourse do not have much of a change in their hymens.

The vagina connects with the uterus, or womb, at the *cervix* (which means neck). The cervix has strong, thick walls. The opening of the cervix is very small (no wider than a straw), which is why a tampon can never get lost inside a girl's body. During childbirth, the cervix can expand to allow a baby to pass. The *uterus* is shaped like an upside-down pear, with a thick lining and muscular walls. In fact, the uterus contains some of the strongest muscles in the female body. These muscles are able to expand and contract to accommodate a growing fetus and then help push the baby out during labor. When a woman is not pregnant, the uterus is only about three inches (7.5 centimeters) long and two inches (5 centimeters) wide. At the upper corners of the uterus, the *fallopian* tubes connect the uterus to the ovaries. The ovaries are two oval-shaped organs that lie to the upper right and left of the uterus. They produce, store, and release eggs into the fallopian tubes in a process called *ovulation*. Each ovary measures about one and one-half to two inches (4 to 5 centimeters) in a grown woman.

There are two fallopian tubes, each attached to the side of the uterus. The fallopian tubes are about four inches (10 centimeters) long and about as wide as a piece of spaghetti. Within each tube is a tiny passageway no wider than a sewing needle. At the other end of each fallopian tube is a fringed area that looks like a funnel. This fringed area wraps around the ovary but doesn't completely attach to it. When an egg pops out of an ovary, it enters the fallopian tube. Once the egg is in the fallopian tube, tiny hairs in the tube's lining help push it down the narrow passageway toward the uterus.

The ovaries are also part of the endocrine system because they produce female sex hormones, such as estrogen and progesterone. (The *endocrine system* is the system of glands, each of which secretes different types of hormones directly into the bloodstream, some of which are transported along nerve tracts to regulate a woman's body.

The Purpose of the Uterus

All pregnant mammals carry their developing babies inside their *uterus*. In women this organ is about three and one-half inches long prior to conception of a new fetus—the size of a small pear—and weighs approximately three ounces The lower portion of the uterus is called the *cervix*, which has an opening called an *os*. The os dilates, or expands, to 10 cm in diameter during labor. This allows the head of the baby to push out of the uterus, through the birth canal, and out of the mother's body.

Its function

There are three layers that make up the wall of the uterus. The outer wall is the *serosa* which contains fibers to support the organ. Next is the *myometrium*. This layer contracts during a woman's period to force the inner-most layer, the *endometrium*, to be expelled as a bloody discharge through the vagina. Each month a new endometrium layer forms and thickens so that if the woman conceives a child, it can receive the fertilized egg which must be implanted in the endometrium to survive.

Its significance

The human uterus connects to each of the two ovaries by a fallopian tube. Girls are born with approximately 400,000 eggs already stored in their ovaries. After she reaches puberty, once each month an egg is released into one of her fallopian tubes. Sexual intercourse releases male sperm cells into the woman's body and conception may occur if the sperm and egg meet inside the fallopian tube. Then, stimulated by the hormone progesterone, the fertilized egg must travel to and implant itself into the endometrium that lines her uterus. If the fertilized egg does not reach the endometrium, but remains in the fallopian tube, it is known as an *ectopic* pregnancy that can result in the rupture of the fallopian tube causing infertility or even death for the woman.

Benefits

The uterus of a pregnant woman grows to contain *the fetus* (the developing baby). It also holds the *amniotic fluid* in which the baby swims and is cushioned, as well as the *umbilical cord* through which the baby receives nutrition and excretes waste products. The umbilical cord connects the baby to its mother through the *placenta* which is attached to the wall of the uterus.

Very Important Insights

There are many serious health conditions like uterine cancer, fibroids, etc. that can impact a woman's uterus. The surgical procedure that is done to remove the uterus is called a *hysterectomy*. Over 600,000 hysterectomies each year are performed in the United States, making it the second most common surgical procedure for women.

> Cancer or *fibroids* (benign tumors) that are present in the uterus are found in the *myometrium* lining, the area that houses the fetus. The fetus will be attached to the little white band, which is the lining of the uterus where it begins to grow. It is like a little blanket made and prepared to carry a child. During menstruation this *blanket* sloughs off. The fallopian tubes enter into the uterus, the vaginal canal. During intercourse several hundred million sperm are released into the vagina and travel through the vaginal canal which sits at the mouth of the cervix then enters into the fallopian tube. If conception takes place the sperm penetrates an egg and creates a single set of 46 chromosomes called a *zygote*, which is the basis for a new human being. Fertilization always takes place in the fallopian tube. The fertilized egg then spends a couple of days traveling through the fallopian tube towards the uterus dividing into cells; it is called a *morula*. The morula becomes a *blastocyst* and eventually ends up in the uterus. There it will implant itself and grow into another human being. If there is no intercourse that month, then the existing egg disintegrates after a few days which causes the progesterone hormone level to drop and you begin to see the built up endometrial or sloughing begin.

The Menstrual Cycles—What Really Happens in Those Twenty-Eight Days?

Have you ever wondered about the connection between the twenty-eight day menstrual cycle and the cycle of the moon? Here is a theory: In the days before electricity, women's bodies were influenced by the amount of moonlight seen. All women cycled together. Just as sunlight and moonlight affect plants, animals, oceans, and rivers, levels of moonlight trigger hormones. Today, with artificial light everywhere day and night, our cycles no longer correspond to the moon. As stated previously, if an egg becomes fertilized by a man sperm, pregnancy results and the fertilized egg attaches itself to the woman's uterine wall. If the egg is not fertilized, it will break apart and the thickened lining of the uterus sheds during the menstrual period.

- **Day One** starts with the first day of a woman's period, or menstrual cycle. This occurs after her hormone levels drop at the end of the previous cycle, signaling blood and tissues lining the uterus (womb) to break down and shed from her body. Bleeding lasts about five days.
- Usually by **Day Seven**, bleeding has stopped completely. Leading up to this time, hormones cause fluid-filled pockets, called *follicles* to develop on the ovaries. Each follicle contains an egg.
- Between **Days Seven and Fourteen,** one follicle will continue to develop and reach maturity. The lining of the uterus starts to thicken, waiting for a fertilized egg to implant there. The lining is rich in blood and nutrients.
- Around **Day Fourteen** (in a twenty-eight-day cycle) hormones cause the mature follicle to burst and release an egg from the ovary, a process called *ovulation*.
- Over the next few days, the egg travels down the fallopian tube toward the uterus. If a sperm unites with the egg here, the fertilized egg will continue down the fallopian tube and attach to the lining of the uterus.
- If the egg is not fertilized, progesterone levels will drop around **Day Twenty-Five**. This signals the next menstrual cycle to begin. The egg will break apart and be shed with the next period.

Let's examine the twenty-eighth day when the progesterone level drops causing a breakdown of the endometrial fluid on the lining in the uterus and the period starts to flow. That flow causes the rise in the estrogen hormone which ripens another cell to start the cycle all over again. And then when that cell actually grows, it produces a rise in the estrogen, which is usually seen on the seventh day. Remember, you are beginning to build up to another cycle. The estrogen rises, then two weeks later, the decline in estrogen releases the hormone progesterone which causes the egg cell to break forth. It actually breaks through the thin membrane and leaves a little scar. During ovulation, when the egg breaks out, you may feel a twinge in your side that causes you to double over in pain as if you are having an appendicitis attack. If you check your calendar, you should note that the pain occurs at the midway point between your cycles.

Once ovulation occurs, the scar that is left on the ovary where the egg has burst forth produces progesterone. As the progesterone level rises, the lining of the uterus thickens preparing the uterus to receive the fertilized egg. It acts like a little blanket nestling the little egg for nine months. The progesterone level remains high throughout the nine months of pregnancy. If there is no fertilized egg, the progesterone level drops off and the cycle starts all over again. When the progesterone level drops, there is also a release of a chemical called *prostaglandin*, and that is what causes what has been described as *cramps*. Cramps, or the wave-like motions felt by some women, actually is the increase in prostaglandins causing the muscle to clamp down in the lower abdomen, thighs, and lower back as it tries to move out the thick lining produced by the progesterone.

Chapter Three

THE EMOTIONAL AND NUTRITIONAL NEEDS OF THE ADOLESCENT GIRL

Adolescent Girls Need Dependable Parents

In most instances, adolescent girls go through enormous changes from the internal pressures brought on by the sudden onslaught of chemical and psychological changes and from external peer and family pressures.

Biological changes, the rejection of her parents and their standards, a preoccupation with the opposite sex, all are factors that literally underlie most of their behavior. They are just a ball of confusion and they cannot explain to you what is going on. If asked, "What's going on with you today? Why can't you keep still?" she would not know how to respond. Just understand that this is a phase and that she is going to come out okay.

She does not need to be punished for every seeming violation of parental values, unless there has been a real breach in her behavior. Parents may need to develop some level of comfort with displays of resistance from their daughters and not confront every little flinch she makes. When I say resistance, however, I don't mean all out anarchy. She should not be allowed to run your home. Your adolescent may say things like, "Aw, Ma, shut up, don't talk to me!" This type of attitude should not be tolerated, but don't make her march like a little soldier or automaton. Give her room to explain what she is feeling. If she is out of control, get the help of a professional. Schedule an appointment with a local family therapist.

Part of being acceptable to her peers is to be unacceptable to her parents. If an adolescent girl is to be accepted by her peers, she feels she must leave some parental values behind and also those of her teachers and other adults. So if her peers say, "Let's do this," although the she knows it's wrong, she will do as her peers say. Anything that her parent says is wrong. She will do the opposite of whatever they say. If her Mom says she likes what she is wearing, she will go and change her clothes. She may start using obscene language, begin smoking, or experimenting with drugs. She may even become sexually active (sometimes with the same sex), as a way of self-experimentation and out of boredom. During counseling, girls sometimes admit they did not pick up the habit of swearing from their parents, but rather they picked it up in the streets and do it because it makes them feel important and accepted by their peers. This is the time of your daughter's life when she wants to share her thoughts and feelings with someone her own age. Parents should not get nervous over it. Just correct the unacceptable behavior. Anger muddies the atmosphere, so losing one's temper is unproductive.

From infancy, an open and unguarded environment must be set in place in the home so that during the turmoil of adolescence, she will have something that is stable to rely on. She may be going through adolescence at the same time her mother is going through her own mid-life crisis. The husband may feel as though he is the only sane person in the house. The daughter actually wants to try to spread her wings and discovers that there is more to life outside than what she is accustomed to at home. This is the natural course of independence. In this process, she will discover that not all acquaintances are good for her. This is when parents need to be adaptable to her thoughts and feelings and make sure the doors of communication are wide open so she feels free to talk to you about things that are happening in her life. The most likely places that she will make positive relationships with friends will be through the things that she likes to do—sports, dance, church and school choir, and other extracurricular activities where friends share a common goal together. These types of relationships are healthy and necessary for her development. They provide support and encouragement to adolescents during these confusing years. It is also important to remember that other adults who demonstrate ongoing commitment and care play an essential role in a girl's development. Conversely, the lack of a close, caring adult during adolescence could interrupt or delay her development. Without a close adult, and without confidence in her own judgment or abilities, she may be more likely to turn to her peers for support and validation more often than she should. Although research about delinquency among girls is still scarce, some researchers are focusing on a "developmental pathway to delinquency" (Belknap & Holsinger, 1998).

Just as girls and boys develop in different ways physically and emotionally during adolescence, their pathways to delinquency are often gender specific. The problems faced by girls and young women can be viewed as part of a developmental continuum linking early problems (such as family dysfunction, abuse, loss of a primary caregiver, and other traumas) to later behavioral problems (Oregon Commission on Children and Youth Services, 1990). During the teen years, when girls are transitioning to adulthood, unresolved issues from earlier stages of their development may come to a head. Incomplete bonding in infancy, sexual abuse in childhood, failed relationships with adults, and other problems can result in an inability to form positive relationships, lack of self-respect, ignorance of physical health and sexuality issues, and low self-image (Oregon Commission on Children and Youth Services, 1990). Substance abuse at a young age can also interrupt a girl's psychosocial development. As one researcher observed, "It is not unusual to have a 16-year-old check into a residential drug treatment program with both her works' (needle and syringe) and a well-worn stuffed animal hidden in her backpack." (Acoca, 1995).

So, how do you stay in the loop of an adolescent woman's life without stepping over her newly created boundaries of trust and growth? Here are some tips:

- Stay involved with her activities in school and elsewhere. Know where she is at all times and lend a hand with any organization that allows parent involvement, which is most of them.
- Check homework regularly. Dropping grades can be sign of anxiety and may need to be corrected by getting to the bottom of the problem.
- While a girl of this age may argue about clothes she is allowed to wear out of the house, look for drastic changes in styles, as this could be a sign of bad peer pressure dictating what is in style.
- Let her know that you love her regularly, give her some space, and when she does want to talk, listen intently (without talking or criticizing unless it is necessary).

Adolescent girls need dependable parents. They need to count on parents' presence and support as they test their personal limits. Her testing of personal limits is a requirement for identity formation. It demands that she should be able to push against a reasonably healthy and solid person. I remember my daughter as a toddler first venturing out into exploration and autonomy, but she needed a mother figure to be there. She wanted to do things on her own, but wanted her mother to be nearby. She needed to find her boundaries and self-identity within the limits of safety. This held true for her all the way through her adolescence. Now suppose one of the parents is needy and wants the daughter to show how grateful she is for all he or she has done for her. In that instance, the adolescent daughter has to interrupt her identity formation to take care of the needy parent. The need for dependency is the need for predictability and meaning. Children need their parents to be there for them in a reasonable and predictable manner. In chronically dysfunctional families, the children never know what to expect. The father may always be drunk and not be at home. The mother may be hysterical or a hypochondriac. The children have to walk on eggshells. They never know what is coming next. The "rageaholic" father may have an outburst at the most unexpected times. When the fathers have an emotionally distant relationship with their wives, they, as a consequence turn to their adolescent daughters for care, intimacy, and affection. Quite often the daughters suffer with depression, anxiety, and low self-esteem. Girls with healthy self-esteems are realistic and generally optimistic. In contrast, girls with low self-esteem can find challenges to be sources of major anxiety and frustration. Those who think poorly of themselves have a hard time finding solutions to problems. If given to self-critical thoughts such as "I'm no good" or "I can't do anything right," they may become passive, withdrawn, or depressed. Faced with a new challenge, their immediate response might be, "I can't."

> *If there be righteousness in the heart, there will be beauty in the character.*
> *If there be beauty in the character, there will be harmony in the home.*
> *If there be harmony in the home, there will be order in the nation.*
> *If there be order in the nation, there will be peace in the world.*
>
> *By Sathya Sai Baba*

Is Your Self-Esteem Reflecting In Your Daughter?

Loving your daughter through her self-esteem issues

The doorway to your daughter's social and mental health is planted in her self-esteem. Simply put, it is how she feels about herself. This word is the foundation of her well-being and the key to her success as an adult. Regardless of her age, how she feels about herself affects her inter and intra personal life and determines how she acts and reacts to the people around her. It is important for you to help her build her self-esteem. Giving her a real positive sense of herself comes with lots of positive praise and reinforcement.

Her self-esteem is how she perceives herself

It is not enough for her to be able to look in the mirror and like the person she sees, for that only gives her a shallow image of herself. But, when she is able to look inside herself and feel comfortable with how she feels, she becomes empowered with a healthy self-esteem. How she feels about herself can have a profound effect on her physical and emotional health. Girls, who constantly see themselves and their life in a negative light, work themselves into a state of low self-esteem and depression.

A lack of a healthy self-image often leads to behavior problems

The majority of behavioral problems I've encountered in counseling come from poor self-worth in parents as well as children. Why is one person a delight to be with, while another always seems to drag you down? How people value themselves, get along with others, perform at school, achieve at work, and relate in marriage, all stem from the strength of their self-esteem.

Does a healthy self-esteem mean being narcissistic or arrogant?

No, it means having a realistic understanding of her strengths and weaknesses. She enjoys her strengths and has the wisdom to work on her problem areas. Because there is such a strong parallel between how a person feels about herself and how a person acts, helping your daughter to build self-confidence is vital to discipline.

Throughout your daughter's life she will be exposed to influence builders (positive people) and influence breakers (negative people). Your responsibility as her parents is to expose her to more builders and help her to work through the breakers.

Be her best cheerleader

I realize that it can be very challenging to find the time and motivation to always compliment your daughter when she does the right things. We often get caught up in our own day-to-day life and forget to offer praise or an admiring comment to our children when they try. But these small gestures, "I am very proud of you. You are very special to me," can change the energy in your home and your relationship with your daughter. You are the molder of her dreams. You can break or build her future endeavors by the things you say and do. Her very life depends on you. If you are vibrant and happy, chances are, she will be also. You are her first and most visible role model. You are the first to tell her who she is as a person with or without saying a word. Modeling healthy emotional values is the best way to build your daughter's self-esteem.

Some teenage girls have very poor images of themselves. They sometimes confuse body image with self-image. So be careful what you're modeling for her. She may look like you, so if she watches, as you look at yourself in the mirror, and your response is, "I look terrible. I am so fat, I hate the way I look in this dress!" You have just modeled for her a person with some form of low self-image. The idea of a perfect body for some girls comes directly from individuals they admire most, such as models in magazines or TV. If these girls don't think they resemble their idols and they have poor body image, then their self-image also suffers. Make sure you are conscious of modeling healthy self-acceptance and self-confidence in your own life. So, cheer her on even if you are convinced that her wanting to be a singer is not her gift; and she is not going to be the next Beyonce! Don't discourage her. Allow her to discover for herself that singing is not her gift and that she may have to explore several other activities and may fail a few times before she finds her true gift.

Identify and redirect inaccurate beliefs

It is imperative that you help your daughter to have a healthy and accurate belief system about herself and the world around her. She may need to have a paradigm shift, or what is sometimes called an *"Aha"* moment, when the composite picture in her mind is experienced in another way. We all have internal dialogue or conversations with and about ourselves that include all of our life experiences. Whether these experiences are based on truth or are completely false, your daughter may feel that no one likes her because

33

she has had several experiences by people who did or did not like something she did. Because of this, she associates this experience with not being lovable. If she then encounters someone who showers her with love, she may push him or her away because negative self-talk will convince her that she is unattractive and therefore unlovable. To combat this negative self-talk, she would have to adapt an internal dialogue that says, "I am going to accept myself. I'm going to raise the bar to what I expect from myself. I will never go back to where I was." This new internal dialogue can help her to identify and redirect her inaccurate beliefs into a positive and accurate belief system.

Spend what time is necessary each day with your daughter redirecting her belief system whether it concerns perfection, attractiveness, ability, or anything else. Help her to set more accurate standards and become more realistic in evaluating herself. This will help her to have a healthy self-concept. Talk and listen to her or seek professional help when necessary to uproot any inaccurate perceptions she may have of herself and the world around her. If left alone her negative self-concept can take root and become her reality. For example, she might be a wonderful and loving person, but struggle with making friends, so her belief system concludes that she is ugly and not worth being around. Not only is this a false generalization, it is also a belief that can put her future in jeopardy.

Every girl needs to be accepted for who she is. This builds her confidence and her ability to stand her ground when pressured to stray away from her values. Let your daughter know what you admire about her. Encourage her to pursue her own unique interests. Make a conscious effort to understand her, even if you don't agree with her. Teach her how to speak up for herself, even if others disagree with her point of view. Your responsibility is to help her to have a healthy sense of identity so she will be able to assert herself when needed and to see herself as a capable and lovable individual. Don't only tell her but show her that you love and respect her and enjoy her company. Give her special tasks that enable her to feel significant and successful.

Parenting is very therapeutic. In loving your daughter, you show her that you care for her, which often results in your own healing from your past.

Breaking your own parenting pattern of the past

It is important to keep in mind that a child's self-esteem is acquired and not inherited. Certain parenting traits and certain character traits, such as anger and fearfulness, are learned in each generation. Having a child gives you the rare opportunity to become the parent you wish you had. If you suffer from low self-confidence and feel that it is a result of how you were raised, here is an opportunity to heal yourself and escape the family bondage and patterns of the past. You cannot change what you don't acknowledge.

Try this exercise. Therapist calls this "passing on the best, and discarding the rest."

- List five specific things your parents did to build your self-esteem.
- List four specific things your parents did that affect your self-esteem.
- Now resolve to emulate the good things your parents did and avoid the rest. If you find it difficult to follow through with this exercise on your own, get help from a professional. Both you and your daughter will benefit.

It's time to leave mother and father (or home)

Your mom and dad did their best given their circumstances and the prevailing parenting climate of the times. Three generations of mothers, Grandma, Mom and her teenage daughter once visited my office. They were all angry at each other. I remember the grandmother saying to the mother, "I was a good mother to you. I sent you to live with my mother because my husband didn't like you. I sent money every month." The younger mother was angry and resentful of her mother and forbade her teenage daughter to have a relationship with her grandmother. The teenage daughter loved and bonded with her grandmother and resented her mother for not spending anytime with her. She was angry and had very little boundaries. I asked them to take a look at how the pattern of abandonment is followed by anger and resentment when very low self-esteem is followed through the generations.

She sees the reflections in the mirror

None of us can put on a happy face all the time, but as a parent your unhappiness can transfer to your daughter. She looks to you as a mirror of her own feelings. If you are worried, you can't reflect good feelings. In her early years, her concept of self is so intimately enmeshed into her mother's concept of herself that a sort of mutual self-worth building goes on. What image do you reflect to your daughter? She will see through a false facade to the troubled person beneath. Children translate your unhappiness with yourself to mean unhappiness with them. Even infants know they are supposed to please their parents. As they get older, they may even come to feel responsible for their parents' happiness. If you are not content, they must not be good (or good enough). If you are experiencing serious problems with depression or anxiety, seek help so that you can resolve these feelings before they affect your daughter.

Give her positive reflections

Some of her self-image comes not only from what she perceives about herself, but from how she thinks others perceive her. When you give your daughter positive reflections, she learns to think well of herself. She will also willingly rely on you to tell her when her behavior is not pleasing. This becomes a discipline tool. "All I have to do is look at her a certain way and she stops misbehaving," said a mother I once counseled. She had saturated her daughter's self-awareness with what she called "positive feelings," and her daughter was used to the reflection in her mother's face, so much so, that she knew exactly what every look meant.

Your Adolescent Daughter's Nutritional Needs

During her adolescent years, her body goes through a period of rapid growth and maturation when requirements for energy and almost all nutrients are increased. During this period, her eating habits tend to change from her earlier years due to her new found independence from her parent's supervision, increased socialization with peers, part-time work, and the ability to buy food away from home. Adolescents tend to skip meals more often (especially breakfast) than adults. They often have a diet high in sweets, highly processed foods, fried foods and fast foods thus resulting in poor nutrition. Unfortunately, the top sources of calories in a teen's diet include some unhealthy choices: sweets, such as cake and cookies, pizza and soda. A healthier eating plan for the adolescent girl should include more whole natural foods, such as whole grains, fruits, vegetables, lean proteins and low-fat dairy products. She needs three servings of fruits a day, in which one serving is equal to one medium apple or 1 cup of fresh cut-up fruit. Vegetables also make healthy additions to her diet. Like fruits, vegetables are low in calories and rich in essential nutrients that promote health. She needs four servings of vegetables a day. An example of a vegetable serving includes 1/2 cup of cooked vegetables or 1 cup of mixed salad greens. Teen girls can easily meet their daily veggie needs by including them at both the lunch and dinner meal, as well as eating them as a snack. If she does not get the proper nutrients she may have problems in the following areas of her maturation:

- She will most often experience a delay in her physical growth and development.
- Her cognitive development will be affected resulting in lower IQ (lower by 15 points.)
- She will experience a greater degree of behavioral problems now and in her adult life.
- Her sexual maturation and growth would be delayed.
- She will have a decreased attention span. (ADHD)

I realize that these may not be popular statements due to society's high promotion of a low calorie diet; however, most adolescent girls need to maintain a high caloric way of eating to maintain an appropriate level of energy. The amount of calories she takes in is not the problem but rather it is the kinds of food that the calories derive from. An adolescent girl needs approximately 2,000 calories each day. She also needs to maintain a healthy amount of other nutrients such as calcium, proteins, and iron, as well as fats and oils.

Whole-Grains

Most teens get enough grains in their diet but not enough whole grains, according to the U.S. Department of Agriculture. Whole grains are high in fiber and a natural source of iron, magnesium, selenium and B vitamins. Fifteen-year-old girls need five to eleven servings of grains a day, and at least half of those grain servings should be whole-grain. One whole grain serving equals two slices of whole wheat bread or 1 cup of cooked brown rice.

Vitamin D for Bone Health

To keep her bones strong and prevent osteoporosis later in life, she needs to make sure she gets enough calcium and vitamin D in her diet. Dairy foods are a good source of both and the adolescent girl needs three servings a day, in which one serving is equal to 1 cup of low-fat milk or one small carton of low-fat yogurt.

Energy Requirements

Every adolescent has a great need for energy in order to have proper growth and for any activity she may be involved in. The energy requirements for an adolescent girl varies depending on age, body size, activity levels. In many respects, the nutrients and energy needs of an adolescent are higher than those of any other age group. A healthy adolescent have large appetites and it is important that they eat food of high nutritional value in the form of a well-balanced meals rather than too many snacks that are rich in fat, sugar or salt. To meet her nutritional requirements, she should choose a variety of healthy foods, such as lean proteins, low fat, some dairy products, fruits, vegetables and nuts. It is important that she avoids unhealthy foods high in fat, particularly saturated fats and/or sugar, both at home and at school.

Water

The adolescent girl should think of water as a very important part of her nutrition. Hydration is important for maintaining body fluids and minerals, such as sodium. This stands true especially if she is a physically active young lady. She may need more water than her sedentary counterparts due to fluid loss through sweat. Water serves many functions in the human body. It serves as the medium in which metabolic reactions occur. Water helps lubricate joints, cushion organs and regulate body temperature. You need water in large quantities daily; and it is important for food digestion, proper absorption of nutrients and waste removal. The requirement for water is expressed as "total" water—which includes all water contained in food, beverages and drinking water. Your body needs approximately seven cups daily.

Physical Activity

Regular physical activity is important for anyone's health, particularly adolescents. Not only is it going to help the development of bone strength, but muscle mass is going to increase. Several studies have shown that there are other significant benefits of exercising a couple of hours every week. It is important to therefore encourage your adolescent daughter to take up a sport in her school or community. She can also engage in other physical activities to protect her bones and improve her overall health for many years.

Fats and Oils

It is imperative that fats be a part of the adolescent's diet. Dietary fat plays a very important role as an energy source, a significant cell structural component, and a precursor to agents of metabolic function and a potent gene regulator. I realize that fats have received a bad reputation over the last decade, resulting in a plethora of low-fat diets and fat-free food products. Although certain types of fats or excessively high amounts of fats can be unhealthy, fats are vital to the body. They are essential components of all body tissues and are especially important in the development of cell membrane, the retina and brain tissue. Your body requires fats and oils to support proper growth and development, especially during the adolescent stage. There are two essential fatty acids and alphalinolenic acids. Since the two essential fatty acids cannot be produced by the body, it is required that they be transmitted through foods. When these are missing or deficient in an adolescent's body, it results in growth faltering, skin and vision concerns.

Not all fats are the same, so you should try to avoid:

- Saturated fats, such as butter, solid shortening and lard. These saturated fats are found mostly in foods from animals and some plants. Saturated fats include beef, veal, lamb, pork, poultry, cream, milk, cheeses, and other dairy products.
- Foods from plants that contain saturated fat include coconut oil, palm oil, kernel oil (sometimes called tropical oils) and also cocoa butter.
- Trans fats. These are found in vegetable shortenings, margarines, crackers, cookies, snack foods, and other food made with or fried in partially hydrogenated oils.

If possible use oils such as olive, safflower, sesame, or sunflower. Keep in mind that eating too much fat will put on pounds. Fats have twice as many calories as proteins or carbohydrates.

Proteins

Protein is an important component of every cell in her body. Protein is required for maintenance of existing lean body mass and the development of additional lean body mass during the adolescent growth spurt. Her hair and nails are mostly made of protein; the body utilizes protein to build new and to repair existing tissues, to make enzymes, hormones, and other body chemicals. Proteins are important building blocks of bones, muscles, cartilage, skin and blood. Along with fat and carbohydrates, protein is a macronutrient. This means that the body needs relatively large quantities of it, as compared to vitamins and minerals, which are needed in relatively small quantities and are called micronutrients. However, unlike fat and carbohydrates the body does not store protein, and therefore has no reservoir to draw from when needed for a new supply. Don't assume that your adolescent should be eating protein all day! The fact is that she is probably getting enough proteins from the foods she is presently eating. It has been said that we need more protein to build bigger muscles. The truth is the only way to build bigger muscles is through exercise. Taking large amounts of protein would not increase one inch of your muscles.

Your adolescent daughter need between 45 and 60 grams of protein each day. Most teens easily meet this requirement with their intake of beef, pork, chicken, eggs, and dairy products. Protein is also available from certain vegetable sources, including tofu and other soy foods, beans, and nuts. These foods should be included in the diets of vegetarians especially. When protein intakes are consistently inadequate, reductions in linear growth, delays in sexual maturation and reduced accumulation of lean body mass may occur.

Calcium

Approximately one half of the total body calcium is created or developed during the female adolescent stage. Calcium needs during adolescence are greater than they are in either childhood or adulthood because of the increased demand for skeletal growth. Since calcium is the main mineral that strengthens bones, it is then necessary that she take an adequate amount of calcium. It is essential for the development of strong and dense bones during her growth spurt. Inadequate calcium intake during adolescence and young adulthood puts her at risk for developing osteoporosis later in life. In order to get the required 1,300 milligrams of calcium, she is encouraged to consume three to four servings of calcium-rich foods each day. Milk should provide the greatest amount of calcium in her daily nutritional regiment, next green leafy vegetables, followed by cheese, ice cream and frozen yogurt.

Iron

An adolescent gets less than sixty percent of the recommended daily iron intake although it is vital for transporting oxygen in the bloodstream. So most adolescents are iron deficient. As the adolescent girl gain muscle mass, more iron is needed to help her new muscle cells obtain oxygen for energy. The onset of menstruation also imposes additional needs for more iron. It is recommend that her daily intake of iron be approximately 12-15 mg per day.

Iron Deficiencies

Many adolescents may have iron deficiency anemia-a decrease in the number of RBCs in her body and not necessarily have any signs or symptoms because the body's iron supply is depleted slowly. But as the anemia progresses, some of these symptoms may appear:

- Fatigue and weakness, pale skin, rapid heart beat, irritability, decreased appetite, dizziness or a feeling of lightheadedness

Good sources of iron include beef, chicken, pork, fish, boiled or poached egg, legumes (including beans), enriched or whole grains, and leafy green vegetables, such as spinach or dried figs.

Zinc

Zinc is an essential mineral for the adolescent girl. It stimulates the activities of approximately one hundred enzymes in her body.

- It supports her immune system.
- It is necessary to synthesize her DNA.

- It essential for healing her wounds.
- It supports growth and development during her growth spurt and beyond.

Zinc is present in a variety of our daily foods, such as red meat, poultry, whole grains, fortified cereals, beans, nuts and dairy products. Because of the rapid growth and hormonal changes during adolescence, the serum zinc level has a tendency to decline in response to these rapid changes. For adolescent females ages 14-18, the RDA recommends 9 mg per day. Zinc is naturally abundant in red meats, shellfish, and whole grains. Additionally, many breakfast cereals are fortified with zinc. Zinc and iron compete for absorption, so elevated intakes of one can reduce the absorption of the other. Adolescents who take iron supplements may be at increased risk of developing mild zinc deficiency if iron intake is over twice as high as that of zinc.

Zinc Deficiencies

- Growth retardation, diarrhea, hair loss, delay in sexual maturation, impotence, loss of appetite, lesions of the eyes and skin, and white spots on the fingernails

Folate

Folate is a part of the Vitamin B family. It plays a vital role in DNA (which tells the cells what it will be and how it will work), RNA, and protein synthesis. Thus, adolescents have increased requirements for folate during puberty. It is needed in the body for:

- Making red blood cells. They carry oxygen to all parts of the body. Healthy red blood cells help her to have energy for her daily activities.

Folate Deficiencies

Isolated folate deficiencies are uncommon. A deficiency of folate usually co-exists with other nutrient deficiencies because of its association with a poor diet. However, you may see symptoms similar to that of anemia, such as:

- Weakness, fatigue, difficulty concentration, irritability, headache, heart palpitations, shortness of breath

Rich sources of dietary folate for adolescent girls include ready-to-eat cereal, orange juice, bread, milk, and dried beans or lentils. Adolescents who have formed the habit of skipping breakfast or do not include orange juice and ready-to-eat cereals in their meals may be at an increased risk of low folate consumption.

Chapter Four

THE STAGES OF THE ADOLESCENT GIRL'S DEVELOPMENT

Let's take a look at how the adolescent stages unfold. Adolescence is a challenging period for both children and their parents. The three stages of adolescence—early, middle, and late—are experienced by most teens, but the age at which each stage is reached varies greatly from child to child. These different rates of maturation are connected to physical development and hormone balance, neither of which the child can control. For this reason, adolescents should be treated as individuals and any guidelines should be adapted to the particular child.

Early Adolescent Girl (11-13 Years)

The Eleven-Year-Old

Eleven year-olds differ somewhat in their development than ten year-olds. Eleven year olds may exhibit loud, assertive, moody and selfish behavior that was not present in earlier years. They tend to object to every little request. *"Do I have to?"* They whine and sing it. They interact better with outsiders than they do with their own parents. They will honor the requests of others, but will not reciprocate if asked to do something at home. Most requests at home are followed by complaints like, "Goodness, why can't *she* do it! I'm always being told to do things." During this time you need to give her some flexibility. She needs space with boundaries, just enough to let her know that she has room to turn, but she doesn't have room to control your home.

A girl's appetite changes when she turns eleven. She may either eat everything in the refrigerator or nothing at all. Eating disorders, such as bulimia and anorexia nervosa, can occur at this age if they are insecure and are pressured to straighten up their act. These eating disorders and her biological changes are simultaneous. She craves food of any kind, gobbles it down quickly, but then looks at her body and says, "Oh my God, I put on a pound!" Then gags herself and throws it all back up. This is when she starts trying to become "perfect." This need for perfection usually comes from her being compared to some other girl she and her parents may both know. Her self-esteem is fragile and needs to be pampered. The need to control her own life is very important to her. Parents should not encourage this idea of perfection by adding pressure of any kind—teasing about baby fat, commenting on weight gain/loss or comparisons to others. These behaviors are inappropriate and can lead to a quick onset of eating disorders.

The Twelve-Year-Old

The twelve-year old's world is a bit more relaxed. They are beginning to mellow out a tiny bit and are a bit more tolerant of their parents. She is more enjoyable to be around. Do not expect her to volunteer to do work, but she will be a bit more cooperative if you ask her to do things. She will be very insecure about school, especially if she is beginning to grow little breast buds. If her breast buds came too soon, she is upset; if they haven't come at all, she will be upset. Just be open-minded with her and aware of what is going on in her life. Depending on how fast she develops, her menstrual cycle may begin at this time. If she is not starting her cycle, she may feel left out. Or if she started too soon ahead of her peers, she may feel awkward. She may still play with her dolls; this type of behavior shows that she is not emotionally ready for the biological changes that are occurring. Her mind has not caught up with her body at this time. Twelve-year-olds that appear to be restless may need to begin extra-curricular activities. Soccer, swimming or some other sport of her choosing may help to release some of this trapped energy in her body. Quite often this pent up energy is quite sexual in nature; she may be totally unaware of it, but it is quite real.

As a parent you need to focus on saving your authority for the main issues, as to whether or not they can date, appropriate curfews, etc. Avoid nit picking at every little thing. Releasing your child to grow is very important for her future development. The methods used to release her, as well as the covering given to her afterwards, are equally important. You don't know where they are emotionally, but neither does she. She may want to cuddle or she may want her space. You have to realize that she is just a child.

The Thirteen-Year-Old

Thirteen-year-olds are very similar to twelve-year-olds, just a bit less communicative. Don't worry about it. She is a teenager now. You do not need her approval to be there for her, even though she may rebuff you and say she does not need you. Kissing, hugging, or talking to parents is awkward for her. She is self-conscious, moody, and uncommunicative. Parents may want to say, "I just don't like you." If her father is in the home, this is the time she will begin to divest herself from her mother and move toward her father. If the father lives at home, she thinks her mother is clueless and doesn't know very much. A wise mother puts her pride aside and allows her daughter to believe that daddy knows best, and that is very natural at this stage of her daughter's life. She might even compare herself with her mother by asking her father, "Which one of us is prettier?" or "Who do you love more, Daddy? Do you love me or do you love Mommy?" A wise father should reply by stating, "I love you both. I love your mom with all my heart. She is the one that I chose to love and help me on this journey, and you are a beautiful product of our love. You, however, are my precious little angel, you're my princess." This helps to build their self-esteem. Sometimes, however, the father mistakes this gesture as some kind of sexual come on and molestation occurs.

If the mother did not handle this stage of her life well and suffers from low self-esteem, she may compete with her daughter for her husband's affection. If a girl has been given gender identification by her father who has approved and validated her life, she will be secure in her own body and she will not need another male to try to validate her. She will seek from life that to which she is accustomed. It is through the father that she will find gender identity. How a girl feels about herself comes from how and what her father (or father substitute) feels (or didn't feel) about her and shares with her. Whatever you feel about yourself is because your father paid you compliments or if you have very low self—esteem about who you are as a woman, it is because he did not. Gender identity only comes through the male; this is true for young males and young females. If the father is missing from the home—physically or emotionally—the adolescent girl will choose a male on her own to give her gender identity. The problem is that most of the time the male that she chooses will not give her what she needs, but rather what he thinks she needs with no regard for her emotional and physiological growth. Usually it comes in the form of sex, which confuses her real needs. This also accounts for the constant rise in teenage pregnancies.

It's a fact that children learn vicariously by observing the behavior of others and noting the consequences of their actions. They watch what happens to family members when they succeed or fail and those experiences become a reference for how they live. This is known as modeling. A child is like a computer. They will only put out the data that has been put in them. If there has been no data put in them; nothing comes out. Or if there has been wrong data put in them, wrong data comes out and that is what they feel.

Women who have not been validated or given gender identity at that this crucial time in life, usually try to find men that will treat her the way she feels on the inside. If she feels worthless then she will find men who will treat her that way, validating her, allowing her feelings to become her reality. No validation yields low self-esteem. It is important to understand that you have only twelve years to impact and make the difference in your child's life. After that, she is on her own to live out all of your training and influence from the past twelve years whether good or bad.

The Science of Gender Identity

The gender of every embryo is determined by the father. It is not biologically possible for a woman to choose the gender of her child. In a woman's genes, the eggs will only carry X chromosomes. A man genetically carries both X and Y chromosomes. If there is a Y chromosome in the sperm that fertilizes the woman's egg, the woman will conceive a male baby. If the sperm contains an X chromosome, the woman will give birth to a baby girl. When a man reaches a climax, he ejaculates roughly 1.2 billion sperm cells into the female cervix. The sperm that is released can contain either an X or Y chromosome. No matter how high the sperm count, your eggs can be fertilized with a single sperm.

God gives mothers the ability to carry a child, but only the father can call that child forth, and crown that child with honor by telling him or her, "You are finally a woman, my daughter," or "You're finally a man, my son." Why? Because he has taken his time to do the training through a rites of passage. It takes a father (or a father substitute) to do it. Yes, your child will grow up fine and become an adult male or female without this, but they will always lack gender identity. A woman cannot give gender identity to her children. It takes a male to do it.

The Middle Adolescent Girl (14-16 years)

The Fourteen-Year-Old

At fourteen, young girls begin to settle in a bit and become more assured of themselves. With her new self-assurance comes more rebellion; she is more open and vocal in her behavior. She will be more prone to have outbursts of anger. These outbursts should not be taken personally, although you may feel as though you have lost all control of her. She may say unkind things like, "I hate you! I wish Aunt Keisha and Uncle Mike were my parents. I hate it here!" Respond by telling her that it is alright. She will probably respond, "Whatever!" Try to understand; don't get capsized by her anger. It's okay if she hates you for a spell. Her outbursts will only last for a day or so, or maybe just fifteen minutes! It's not really about you. It's really about her. To compound fears even more, she might also show interest in older boys because to her younger boys are silly at this time. Just ask yourself, "What would Jesus do in this situation?" and be patient! She may rebel against the idea of family counseling, but suggest it any way. She is coming into her own and as the year progresses you will see a shift in her personality. When she cools down, take some time to pray with her. God will give you the temperament to deal with her outbursts. He knows that she will eventually get it together, because He knows her heart.

The Fifteen and Sixteen Year-Old

At age fifteen, there will be a transition from play and fun to a more serious approach to her new endeavors. As the year goes by, she will begin to earn your trust as her parents. Instill trust and faith in her by giving her responsibilities. She will take pride in her accomplishments and gain poise. She will spend more time alone, listening to music on her iPod, texting friends on her iPhone, doing homework, watching TV or reading. She has a need to be alone more mentally as she is beginning to know herself more deeply.

When a girl turns sixteen, she may start to date, if this is the age you have allowed it, and will begin to relate to you on an adult level. At school she will do things for her teacher, taking on responsibilities. She may be the president of the student council. She feels more responsible. She believes she understands what you feel now and you can talk to her in an adult manner. Her thinking has moved from concrete to abstract. She thinks more about eternal things like God, heaven, hell, and salvation.

Keeping Order in Your Home Without Losing Your Daughter

How do you keep your home from getting out of control during your daughter's adolescence? 1) Maintain control by understanding that what she is going through is necessary and healthy for her future adult life. 2) Expect some rebellion and know that some rebellion is necessary. If guided by your healthy parental practice, it will be temporary and purposeful.

The Scripture states that: ". . . rebellion is as the sin of witchcraft, and stubbornness is as iniquity and idolatry. (I Sam. 15:23) This, however, is not the type of rebellion of which I speak. I am not talking about willful disobedience. I am talking about frustration in the young adolescent who doesn't know what they are doing and are unsure whether they will ever come out from behind the rock and hard place they are in. They don't understand the biological and emotional changes that are taking place in their bodies. Not knowing what to do, they pull away from their parents and situations that nurtured and brought comfort to them in earlier years in order to wean themselves from it. This pulling away from parents works as a coping mechanism. Allowing your daughter to find and navigate her own way without hurting herself is the type of rebellion that works without breaking any laws. Parents can negotiate with many different styles. The first step is to assess her personality type; that will tell you what type of negotiation approach to take. If she is highly rebellious, you do not necessarily want to approach the negotiations in a heavy-handed way. One of the first steps in training your daughter in negotiation basics is to make sure she can predict the consequences of her actions so she has a sense of responsibility for the outcomes generated.

The five critical steps to successful negotiations with your daughter are:

- Narrow the area of dispute.
- Find out what it is she really wants.
- Work with her to find a middle ground.

- Be specific in your agreement and the negotiation's outcome.
- Make negotiated agreements short-term in the beginning.

Steven Wahlroos, in <u>Family Communication</u>, lists a number of rules to help both adolescents and parents communicate so genuine understanding is achieved.

- Always remember that actions speak louder than words.
- Define what is important and ignore what isn't.
- Be as realistic as possible.
- Be clear and specific.
- Be as positive as possible.
- Check out your assumptions. Recognize that it is alright for two people to view the same thing differently.
- Recognize that you both know each other well.
- Keep discussions from turning into arguments.
- Become aware of and express your true feelings.
- Accept her feelings and try to understand them.
- Be considerate and respectful.
- Do not preach or lecture; ask questions instead.
- Do not use excuses.
- Do not nag, yell, or whine.
- Know when to use humor and when to be serious.
- Above all, listen.

I have found that a list like this is much easier to talk about than it is to follow. It may be a good idea to copy and enlarge this and hang it in a public place for both you and your adolescent to see.

Late Adolescence (17-21 years)

I realize that thousands of early adolescent boys and girls accept Christ as Lord and Savior of their lives. I also realize that after accepting Christ at that very early age, many of them continue doing their own thing for a while. Then, at around age seventeen, salvation becomes very meaningful to them and it is at that point they begin to follow Christ seriously and continue doing so for a lifetime. Several of the young people that I know said that age seventeen was the turning point in their lives; when they finally understood the seriousness of life. So, this is the age that the adolescent moves from the exclusively concrete into the abstract.

The seventeen-year-old girl begins to understand God and make decisions about her spiritual life. To her the world is no longer concrete, it is becoming very realistic and so she is beginning to plan her education beyond high school. She begins to think ahead in terms of pursuing college and deciding what she wants to study. This is also the time the government begins to trust them; they are licensed to drive, they can be drafted and accepted into the Armed Forces, and enjoy other rites of passage into adulthood. As she begins to realize her mortality she worries about and becomes concerned about her future. She takes pride in her work, (some can be self-reliant) and thinks seriously about her career goals.

By seventeen, the majority of changes associated with puberty have already taken place. She is now very concerned with her physical appearance and she believes others are also. Most of her time is invested in grooming, exercising, and experimenting with new images such as makeup and clothing styles. This is done with the purpose of developing a satisfying and realistic body image. There are increased concerns about her sexual attractiveness with a movement towards heterosexuality, in most cases. Curiosity and/or attraction towards the same sex may also occur. Although upsetting to some parents, most of the time it is temporary. Tenderness is shown toward the opposite sex with frequently changing relationships. Sexuality is a major preoccupation for this age group.

This late adolescent stage is very much like exchanging her bicycle for a Kawasaki ZX-14R and telling her not to drive over fifty miles per hour until she is married. Girls use clothes, accessories, and fashion to define themselves. They make statements about their choice of peer groups, and establish their psychological identities. For some, the right outfit can serve as a conduit to a popular clique. For others, clothing choice allows them to fly under the radar. It sometimes might even make the difference between a girl fitting in or opting out of her school community entirely. I believe that girls should dress according to their age, however, this is not about me. Most adolescent girls leave home showing cleavage, belly buttons, and/or butt cheeks. The parochial school around the corner from my office has a uniform dress code yet, after school the girls fold over their waistband several times, shortening their skirts to reveal 80% of their thighs. It is important that these girls know how their seductive attire stimulates the sexual arousal of the adolescent boy. Her need for attention and love coupled with his raging hormones creates the proper environment for sexual experiments.

At this age, her relationship sphere broadens to include adults outside her family. At first she may be frightened and feel somewhat exposed by the new and unfamiliar situations and lifestyles, causing her to worry about separation from friends and peers of earlier years. These separation anxieties may prompt her to journal her inner thoughts and feelings. New friends become everything in her life, so choosing quality friends becomes important. Loss of any of these friendships can cause serious depression. She still has a need for peer approval as she did a year earlier, however, her peers have less influence. A year or so ago she would rather go to the movie or a show with friends, now she prefers to do so one-on-one with the opposite sex. As much as she needs her peers, there is an emergent ability to make independent decisions and to compromise, but she still has a long way to go.

She will still complain that her parents interfere with her independence and sometimes during this stage she will experience the most conflict with her parents because of annoying habits or staying out too late. She feels she is too old and independent to have or abide by curfews. She feels entitled to entertain the opposite sex in her parents' home, may refuse to help with house chores, exhibit poor manners, keep messy rooms, or dress inappropriately when going out.

Your Daughter's First Gynecological Examination

As a girl grows into her teenage years, it is important that she receive appropriate medical care. The American College of Obstetrics and

Gynecology (ACOG) recommends that young women have their first visit with an obstetrician-gynecologist (OB/GYN) between the ages of thirteen and fifteen or when they become sexually active, whichever comes first. For most teens, the first visit will not include a pelvic exam. If your daughter has abnormal vaginal bleeding, painful periods, unusual vaginal secretions, or other problems that may be associated with her reproductive health, however, she may need a pelvic exam.

The idea of seeing a gynecologist or having a pelvic exam can make a girl feel nervous, embarrassed, or scared. By explaining why the visit is necessary, giving your daughter a sense of what to expect, and addressing any questions or fears she might have, you can help her feel more comfortable about this experience. Also, you may want to reassure her that while there are a lot of different parts of the gynecological exam, the entire exam and the part she might feel most uncomfortable about does not take long.

Explaining the Importance of the Exam

Chances are your daughter has associated visits to the doctor with health problems or illness. She may or may not understand why she should go to the doctor when she feels perfectly fine.

Explain that this visit serves at least three main purposes:

1. **Information**—She can obtain accurate information and confidential answers to any questions she may have concerning sex, sexuality, her changing body, and menstruation.
2. **Prevention**—She can learn about pregnancy prevention, sexually transmitted diseases, and healthy lifestyles.
3. **Treatment**—For girls who experience missed periods, pain, or other reproductive problems, the doctor can look into why the problems are occurring and offer treatment.

Chapter Five

STAGE TWO-THE GREAT EXPECTATION AND IDEALS: THE SUPERWOMAN (AGES 25-35) LIFE EXPECTATIONS

"Nobody succeeds beyond his or her wildest expectations unless he or she begins with some wild expectations."—Ralph Charell

"Where there is no vision, the people perish . . ." (Proverbs 29:18)

She has graduated from high school and college, and now with a heart full of expectations and a body full of estrogen she sets out to conquer her future dreams. As she formulates her expectations for her life, is she excited about her bright future or is she facing her future with apprehension and fear? For most young women the future holds too many uncertainties and the fear of what might happens tends to overshadow the ray of light that represents the life they ultimately desire. One of the hardest things for her to do in life is to lift herself from her current circumstance and step up to the level of life that she desires. Her expectations not only determine what is going in her life at present, but it also represents what she is willing to settle for in the future. Expectation is a very powerful emotion and one that very few people ever learn to fully cultivate. Whatever you expect with certainty is what you will invite into your life. Expectation is the emotional state where an idea becomes so real that you feel it even though you cannot hold it yet. The biblical text tells us, *"Now faith is the substance of things hoped for, the evidence of things not seen.*"(Hebrews11:1) Though faith and expectation are not the same, they both work in a similar manner, but expectation precedes faith. Once you expect something then you must have faith that it will be accomplished. Expectation is like an invisible magnet that will attract into your life that which you expect. When you expect something, you activate and engage those parts of your mind and your nervous system that can empower you to think the unthinkable and do the undoable. One of the most powerful ways to cultivate expectation is to develop a very clear vision for your life. At this stage of a woman's life, I recommend that she write a personal mission statement to ensure that she has the correct blueprint for her life. She should be aware, however, that her new found super hormones could give her a false sense of invincibility.

At this stage, I believe a woman should stop and ask herself what it means to be a woman. Numerous books, such as *Why Men Don't Have a Clue and Women Always Need More Shoes,* (Pease), *His Needs, Her Needs* (Harley), and *When Two Become One: A Diamond in the Making* (Morgan) have been written that address this difference in biological gender. Back in the 1950s, when my mother was in her twenties, women knew who they were and appreciated it. They knew the characteristics of womanhood enough to know it was okay to be talkative, feminine, and at times emotional. They knew they were nurturing, sweet, and spiritual. That was the natural characteristic of every woman. They loved being helped by men when a door needed to be opened, when a heavy box needed to be carried, or hurt feelings needed to be soothed. They welcomed it. It was a fact of life then, and mothers passed down that information to their daughters in hopes of helping their children understand the role of womanhood and manhood.

Then entered the 1970s, when women's liberation told everyone that women wanted to be treated like men in work as well as every other aspect of life. Please don't get me wrong. I am all for equal pay for equal work, but there is something to the God-given characteristics of the female human being that remains slighted in our present times.

There are two divine characteristics in particular that are peculiar to women and separate them from men. The first is the ability to bring souls to the earth and the second is compassion, which includes a lot more attributes than most people think. We all know that women are mothers. Women are physically able to create babies for future members of our human race, carry them for nine months, and then deliver them here on earth giving them the opportunity to live here for a period of time. With certain characteristics privileged only to women, they raise their children to become good citizens and good human beings. During the years of Great Expectation and Ideals you have the opportunity to embrace your emotions.

Whether moved by kindness or the impression to help another person, these emotions are all a part of being a woman. These God-given attributes are for you to grasp the wonderful understanding of your true potential. The journey to God-given wisdom is not going to be an easy road, so buckle up!

Most people never even take the time to really determine why God created them and what they want from their created lives. Others do what I call the "hope and pray strategy." They kind of know what they want, but they do not believe they can have it, so they hope and pray that something will happen or come along their life's path to fulfill their desires. Expectation, however, is a completely different mindset. It is a mindset of absolute certainty that can be consciously cultivated. Inherent in *hoping* is a sense of doubt so one always holds two opposing results in mind. To *expect* something is to know definitely it is happening. The mind's focus is riveted on one definite end result. To turn a hope into expectation, doubt and fear must be eliminated. Instead of "seeing" something fail or succeed, see only success. With expectation, all thoughts, words, and actions pertain to having and being exactly what is desired. *Expectation* removes the doubt that is inherent in hoping.

When a mother to be is pregnant she says that she is "expecting." In other words, she knows beyond the shadow of a doubt exactly what is going to happen. Although some of the details are still unclear, she is certain that she will have a baby and not something unknown. On an emotional level she can feel the result because she is expecting it, although she can't see and touch it yet. What you expect for your life is exactly what you can expect to come to you. When you start to expect for your life that which you absolutely desire, your whole mindset turns from an uncertain hoping and wishing to the certainty of expecting. The image you encourage, work toward, and entertain in your mind's eye is what going to come your way.

Do not hope for the best but expect the worse. Cultural conditioning teaches young women and men not to get their hopes up so they can avoid disappointment. Aim as low as possible, everything above that will be a bonus. Right? Wrong! Remember, that which you expect with certainty is what you will get in your life. Break away from the masses on autopilot that just settle for an ordinary life. They are not really happy, but they are not unhappy enough to do something about it. If you want to lift your quality of life to a higher level than what it is at the moment, a raising of expectations is the place to begin. Expectations should be raised of who they are as a person and what they believe they deserve. Expectations elevated to a higher level raise standards, and raised standards are the first step to improving your life.

Attracting The Wrong Men!

Like a recurring nightmare, certain women can't seem to break the cycle of attracting men who are wrong for them. There are women who would enter an arena housing 1,000 men; 999 of them would be good for her and one would make her life a living hell. Somehow out of the thousand, she would pick the one that is bad for her. These women seem to have a penchant for ending up in risky relationships and miserable marriages with loathsome males, but why?

I guess a better question would be, "Why are dishonorable males constantly drawn to these women?" But, since we are talking about women, the question is, "Why are so many women attracted to these men who turn out to be abusers, liars, misogynists, cheaters, money-borrowing fakes, and men who end up ripping out the hearts of these women?"

Why Is She Blaming The Man?

I sat in my office listening to Gail's every word, as she read me the riot act about all of the doggish, filthy, no good men who had hurt her in the past and apparently still are hurting her. Looking at his woman on the surface, you wouldn't have dreamed in a million years that she was a poster girl for failed relationships. She was attractive, well-dressed, a seminary grad with a degree in Psychology and Pastor of a church of approximately four hundred parishioners. Yes, she looked like she had it all together! She ended her male bashing tirade by stating, "If I put all of my worthless ex-boyfriends and husbands together in a room, they still couldn't produce one single solitary good man!" Gail insisted that all men are dogs and blamed all men for her pain. She refused to consider the thought that her recurring love traumas could be her own fault. Usually the duration session is one hour, however, I listened to her for two hours as she described the men that she allowed to cause all this pain and anger in her life. As she described these men, I must say I concurred, they were indeed certified dogs! My questions to her were, "What was your pay-off in choosing these men?" and "Why didn't you recognize the pattern of choosing men who mistreated, used, and abused you?"

The fact is that she allowed these "men" into her life. She permitted them to tamper with her physical body. She also allowed them to toy with her emotions and play with her feelings. It took three sessions before I was able to convince her that she played a part in her own painful dilemma. As she came to grips with this new awareness, her anger and rage seemed to subside a little. Although it was difficult for her, after much soul searching, Gail finally conceded that she had become her own worst enemy. Like many women, she had unwittingly made herself a magnet for such men. Thank God Gail was woman enough to admit it and to do something to rectify her predicament.

So What's A Girl To Do? These Men Will Always Be Around!

Men like this will always be around; they will belittle you, abuse you, lie to you, mislead you, cheat on you, take your money, and be in and out of your life. These men exist only because there is large pool of women who eagerly await the chance to mother these little men. If you are willing to bed them, nurse them, wash their clothes, clean up their mess, and listen to their excuses then you should never complain about the things you permit.

Know The Facts About These Types Of Men

These men learn very early that there are a large number of wounded women out there waiting to enable them by buying their counterfeit affection. They smoothly go from woman to woman leaving a trail of abuse, which includes, but is not limited to: verbal, financial, sexual, physical, and emotional abuse. They pull women in with a promise of love, then the abuse or violence follows. By abusing/hitting women it gives these men a false sense of control, and when that doesn't work, they threaten them with harm.

Be Aware Of Their Deceptions

These men will toy with your emotions and play endless gut-wrenching mind games while at the same time profess their undying love. They will impregnate you and leave you alone in a New York minute! To these men, walking away from kids they sire is just as easy as drinking a glass of water.

These men give a bad name to real men who understand the meaning of what it is to be a man. Real men have a vision for their own lives; they honor, respect, regard, and understand the emotional needs of their women at the highest possible level. They care about their homes, families, and communities. Real men classify these pretenders as proficient connivers and liars. These men have an overarching attitude of entitlement, believing they have special rights to everything they desire without the responsibilities. They justify unreasonable expectations, e.g., your life must be centered around their every need, and when they are caught in a compromising position, they won't admit they are guilty but shift the blame to the woman making her feel guilty.

Some of these men are always coming up with new ways of disrespecting women by displaying their sad behavior in peculiar ways; such as luring unsuspecting women to their apartments, secretly videotaping them while having sex, and then exposing them naked on the internet.

On April 19, 1997 Adam Nossiter, published a report in the New York Times about men who deliberately exposed several women to the deadly HIV virus. One man in particular knowingly exposed 62 women. Thirteen of these women have tested positive for the virus so far. He did not reveal that he was infected to any of his of sex partners. Beware of these types of cases and incidents because they are happening constantly.

Learn To Decipher These Men

It is important to understand the nature of these men that are commonly called "dogs." These men succeed at dogging women who think they are in a relationship with a real man, only to find out later that they are only in an entanglement with a counterfeit man, with animalistic personalities. Like dogs, these "two-legged mutts" shows the same characteristics:

- Dogs pick-up on certain scents
- Dogs detest certain scents
- Dogs mark their territory by urinating or defecating
- Dogs detect the scent left by their predecessors

These men do the same. If you are attracting these kinds of men in your life, you are putting out scents that they are attracted to. Now, if you don't mind being used by these men, stay the course. However, if you are tired of these men, it is time to have a paradigm shift; become an example of how you want to be treated, and start valuing yourself. Do not allow anyone to devalue you.

Do You Value Yourself?

As a woman, the most important insight to gain in life is to value yourself by having a healthy perception of your whole being. This starts by believing that you are a unique, precious, one-of-a-kind, never-to-be-repeated, valuable treasure of God manifested in the flesh. When you don't believe that you are a valuable and worthwhile treasure of God, you send out a strong scent to all dishonorable males that you are worthless and willing to be treated any way they feel. Being a woman of worth and value also means being a woman of purpose who demands respect, love, and honor. A woman of purpose will not respond to the same stimuli as a woman who does not value herself.

"She recognized that her goods were good . . ." Proverbs 31:18

"Who can find a virtuous woman? For her price is far above rubies . . ." Proverbs 31:10

Who can find this unique, precious, valuable treasure of God? Only a rare man is capable of finding her. She is the Proverbs 31 Woman. Believe me, she does exist, but because she is one in a million it takes a special man to find her.

The Proverbs 31 Woman

She is not the average woman. As a matter of fact, the things the average woman does, she refuses to do.

- What the average woman will say, she refuses to say.
- What the average woman wears, she refuses to wear.

- She does not respond to the same kind of man the average woman responds to.
- What makes the average woman bitter, makes this woman of purpose, thoughtful.
- What makes the average woman angry, makes her sweet.
- Her thoughts are different, her motives are different, and her conduct and behavior are also different.
- Every man secretly wishes for this woman of purpose to be in his life but most are not qualified to be in her presence.

Once you realize you are a unique, precious, one-of-a-kind, never-to-be-repeated, valuable treasure of God manifested in the flesh and thus, you are worthy of love, respect and honor; you put out a scent that draws honorable men and repels the dogs.

Sing it from the rooftop, "I am a woman of value and worth!" Don't allow "dogs" to mark you as their territory. Never open up your body, feelings, or emotions to these dishonorable males.

Always Let Your Mate Know How You Need To Be Loved

During this stage, many of you are seeking a partner with whom to spend your life. To have a relationship that really works, loving your partner is not enough. You have to love him exactly how he wants to be loved. Likewise, he must love you the way you need to be loved. This is not a sexual need but an emotional need that we all look for. That is the only way to make a relationship meaningful, by giving and receiving the love that is needed by both of you. Have you taken the time to specifically ask your mate how he wants to be loved? And just as important or even more important, have you let him know how you need to be loved? Don't be afraid, just do it!

Case In Point

A woman visited my office because of failing relationships. She said she believed her previous husband of six years and her current husband both loved her, but she never really felt loved. She always felt empty inside. It seemed to me that both of her husbands loved her from their frame of reference, but not hers. She said she prepared dinner for her current husband each evening, regularly washed their clothes, and never refused him sex (even when she wasn't in the mood). She owned her own home before they met and had no children. From her mate's point of view, none of this was important. After all, he could pay his own mortgage, and cooking meals and engaging in sexually intimate acts are what people in relationships do for each other. She felt, however, that they were not complying with the lists they had made early in their relationship specifying how they wanted to be treated. It was soon revealed that neither of them got to the root of their needs and only dealt with a couple of surface needs. Sooner or later their real needs surfaced and because they were not voiced, their relationship became entangled.

Before a woman can expect her mate to love her how she wants to be loved, she first has to find out her needs. Once she knows how she wants to be loved, the next step is to tell her mate. The key is communication. Most of us are not mind readers. Relationships are a two-way street. Both you and your mate have to love each other the way you each want to be loved. When one person's needs are met and not the other person's needs, resentment develops. Talking openly and honestly about individual needs is vital to the relationship. Sometimes compromise is necessary to experience what Stephen Covey calls a "win-win" relationship. Sometimes you simply cannot give what your mate needs. In my client's previous marriage, independence was the most important thing to her husband, but not to her. She simply could not deal with his independence and he had problems with her smothering. This was a core issue in their relationship. This was an issue that eventually divided them forever.

Love Lesson

1. Before you enter into any relationship, first make a list of how you want to be loved.

2. Commit to sharing this list with your mate (or potential mate) and talk about why the things on the list are important to you.

3. Make sure you follow through and do the things that you committed to do.

4. Always carry yourself with confidence. Hold your head high and never criticize yourself in front of anyone or downplay your talents. For example, if you've invited him to a party that you're hosting, don't criticize your own cooking or the place you call home. Don't constantly talk about the improvements you think you need to make. Instead talk about the things that make you happy, the things about your life you wouldn't change for the world.

5. Take care of your body. Looks are important. There is just no way around that. A man has to be attracted to you physically before he falls in love with you, or is at least willing to spend time with you. If you are not looking your best, or if you think you need to lose those pesky ten pounds, start working out and eat healthily. Do not, however, announce this to him; you don't want to make it seem like you think you aren't good enough for him. Instead, do it quietly albeit with determination. Taking care of your body will do wonders for your confidence, and before long you may have more suitors than you'll know what to do with.

6. Be financially independent. A man will know instantly whether or not you see him as a meal ticket and will drop you like a bad habit. If he's shrewd, he'll dump you right after he has gotten what he wants from you. Like you, no man wants to be used and do not allow any man to use you. Please do not allow any man to borrow money from you at any time, he will not respect you after he gets your cash. Learn to say "No!"

7. Do not talk about commitment on the first date, unless you do not want to have a second date with him. Commitment is something that arises naturally after two people really

get to know each other and are able to recognize how they complement each other's lives. This process cannot be hastened through endless "where is this relationship going" conversations. You can't verbally convince him that he should commit to you. What you can and should do is show him who you are and hope that you two are compatible. If time shows that you aren't compatible, you're actually much better off. Imagine the tears and money you'll save by not going through divorce in the future. Never bring it up first. A man who loves you will be committed to you. It will not be necessary for you to convince him that he should commit to you, he will figure that out on his own. If he doesn't, it's his loss and you should move on.

8. Keep your dates light-hearted and fun. Being with you should seem like a getaway; like a fabulous vacation. He should never dread spending time with you regardless of what you are doing together; be it just spending an evening at home or going out. Don't be clingy and concentrate on yourself, your job, hobbies, friends, and family. Always operate from the premise that you are a catch because you are a gift from God, and there is no one else like you out there.

9. Keep yourself educated and well-informed. Read and keep up with events in the world. If all you can talk to him about is Beyonce, Jay-Z, and reality shows, then you need to expand your horizons. Think about it this way; the country we live in still is at war and is struggling to recover from economic recession, voting rights are being weakened, etc. Be able to carry a conversation on pertinent topics.

Your First Love

For a young woman, giving up your virginity can only happen once in a lifetime. It is not to be taken lightly; it should be a beautiful experience, not just sex. You should not allow your partner to talk you into having sex until you are ready. He will tell you he loves you, whether he loves you or not, and he will promise you the world. Your emotions should be kept at bay; when emotions are involved you are like a lamb going to the slaughter. Remember, you may or may never hear from him again, so you shouldn't play Russian roulette with your feelings. This is meant to be one of the most special times of your life, and should be shared with that one special person. When shared with that special person it will be beautiful and should bring both of you closer together, as close as two souls will ever be. You will be joined, mind, body, and spirit. You will be complete.

The truth of the matter is, the first sexual experience is not always pleasurable. It can be awkward and painful; and not the best experience you will have ever had. If your mate does not treat you with respect, he is not the one to share yourself with. There is nothing you can share with a man that equals that, remember you can only give that part of yourself once. Most couples simply drift apart afterwards, sometimes leaving anger, hatred, and resentment. Most women remember their first sexual encounter as painful or quick. Women that didn't have a good experience with their first encounter would just as soon forget his name. On the other hand, some women did have a great first love and like to remember it and pass it on to their own daughters. Now, just because he was your first love doesn't mean you will want to be with him again. I realize that first loves or relationships with the opposite sex always seem special, and when it doesn't work out hearts are broken, but broken hearts are a part of life's journey.

Never settle for a man who doesn't treat you right. Listen to what others are saying about your relationship; they may not always be right, but the red lights are flashing. If he loves you, he will honor and treat you well by building you up and not tearing you down.

The Childbearing Years

Women will spend approximately one-third of their lives in the childbearing years, a time when they not only have to think about their own health but also the health of the precious lives they are bringing into this world. There are many exciting challenges and wonderful experiences throughout these years. Let me guide you as you journey through some common stages:

- Planning Pregnancy
- During Pregnancy
- Breastfeeding
- High Risk Pregnancy

Healthy Habits for the Childbearing Years

- An overall balanced diet is very important for healthy pregnancies as well as your overall general health. Please consult a competent physician.
- Regular exercise can help overall fitness, heart health, and energy levels.
- If you are exercising regularly before pregnancy, you may be able to continue throughout your pregnancy. It is a good idea to discuss this with your health practitioner first.

Planning Pregnancy

Babies will not always be conceived according to a planned schedule. It is not uncommon for some women to take longer to conceive than planned. This can be discussed with your health practitioner. He or she can help you to learn about your body and the best times to conceive. In the meantime, avoiding smoking, limiting caffeine intake, and adopting an improved diet will help. An overall balanced diet is very important for healthy pregnancies as well as your overall general health. Regular exercise can help overall fitness, heart health, and energy levels before during and after pregnancy. Local Health Fitness Centers usually offer a variety of classes and programs. This should be discussed with your health practitioner. Most couples manage to conceive without a lot of complications. It is important for you to consult your health practitioner for a complete examination when planning your pregnancy or as soon as you find out you are pregnant.

You're Pregnant! What's Next?

Whether your first or sixth baby, pregnancy is an exciting time of changes (there goes that word again!) and new beginnings. Years ago, couples learned about pregnancy and parenting from their extended family of grandparents, aunts, uncles and neighbors sharing their wealth of knowledge and experience. In today's mobile, fast-paced society, we have lost the wisdom of the extended family. It used to be that parents had built-in caregivers, as two or more generations live within the same area. It used to be that parents were able to give on the spot assistance to their children, be it for advice, help, discipline, or day-to-day activities such as feeding, sitting or other parenting concerns. You have to remember that parenting is a learned process and you should tap into your family, friends and community. The statement, "It takes a village," is still awesome and true. Parenting needs supportive communities to provide social and spiritual ties to enhance family growth. When you are involved in a supportive community, your family will grow to its full potential and provide the best environment for children to grow into healthy caring adults. The act of bonding together in a community not only makes our physical and economic life possible, but it brings us to the highest possible spiritual life.

High-Risk Pregnancy

For the most part, the miracle of pregnancy and birth progresses as planned. Some pregnancies, however, are considered high risk and need closer observation and management. These include teenagers under eighteen years of age, women over thirty-five years of age, diabetics, women that have had multiple births, women with current medical problems including eating disorders, or women who have had a previous high risk pregnancy. Your doctor may refer you to a high-risk specialist or a high-risk management center.

Preparing for a Normal Labor and Delivery Process

Congratulations on the impending arrival of your new baby! There have been many months of anticipation and now your baby's due date is near. So what should you expect? Well, your world is about to change, so hold on. Apart from the joy of having a beautiful new member added to your family, in preparation for his or her arrival you can expect the following from the start of labor until the first days with your new baby.

Signs of Labor

The process of giving birth is called *labor.* No one, not even your doctor, can predict with certainty the exact day your labor will begin. Your doctor may give you a due date as a point of reference based on your last menstrual period. Labor is a very unpredictable thing. It can start as early as three weeks before the predicted due date or as late as two weeks after. The following are signs that labor is probably on its way:

- **Lightening**: I do not know why it is called "lightening" however, it occurs in preparation for delivery when your baby's head drops down into your pelvis. Often at this stage your belly may appear to look lower in your abdomen. You may even find it easier to breathe as your baby no longer encroaches on the space allowed for your lungs, but now it may press on your bladder and give you an urge to urinate. Don't be alarmed, this can occur a few weeks to a few hours before the onset of labor.
- **Bloody show**: A small amount of bloody or brownish discharge from your cervix is the released mucus plug that has sealed off the womb from infection. This can occur days before or at the onset of labor.
- **Diarrhea:** Frequent loose stools may sometimes mean labor is imminent.
- **Ruptured membranes or breaking of water:** This is the most known sign that labor is on its way. This is fluid gushing

or leaking from the vagina; it means the membranes of the amniotic sac that surrounded and protected your baby have ruptured. This can occur hours before labor starts or during labor. Most women go into labor within twenty-four hours after this. If labor does not occur naturally during this time frame, doctors may induce labor to prevent infections and delivery complications.

- **Contractions**: It is usual for most expecting women to experience periodic, irregular contractions (uterine muscle spasms) as her labor nears. Contractions that occur at intervals of less than ten minutes are usually an indication that labor has begun.

Stages of Labor

Labor is typically divided into three stages:
Stage 1-The first stage of labor is divided into three phases: latent, active, and transition.

- **The Latent or first phase**: This is the longest and least intense phase. During this phase, contractions become more frequent, helping your cervix to dilate so your baby can pass through the birth canal with ease. Discomfort at this stage is minimal. During this phase, your cervix will dilate approximately three or four centimeters and efface, or thin out. If your contractions are regular, you will probably be admitted to the hospital or birthing center during this stage and have frequent pelvic exams to determine how much the cervix is dilated.
- **The Active or second phase**: During the active phase, the cervix dilates from four to seven centimeters. The pain may be intense at this stage or you may experience pressure in your back or abdomen during each contraction. You may also feel the urge to push or bear down, but your doctor or mid wife will ask you to wait until your cervix is completely open.
- **The Transition or third phase**: This is the phase when the cervix is fully dilated to ten centimeters. Your contractions are

now very strong, painful, and frequent, coming every three to four minutes and lasting from sixty to ninety seconds but seeming more like an hour.

Stage 2-This is the stage when your cervix is completely opened. You will know this when your physician gives you the sign that it is ok to push. Your pushing, along with the force of your contractions, will propel your baby through the birth canal. The fontanels (soft spots) on your baby's head allow it to fit through the narrow canal.

Your baby's head is *crowning* when the widest part of it reaches the vaginal opening. As soon as your baby's head comes out, your doctor will suction amniotic fluid, blood, and mucus from his or her nose and mouth. You will continue to push to help deliver the baby's shoulders and body.

Once your baby is delivered, your doctor, mid-wife, or your partner if he has requested to do so, clamps and cuts the umbilical cord.

Stage 3-Congratulations, your baby is now delivered and is doing well, and you will enter the final stage of labor. In this stage you deliver the *placenta*. The placenta is a membrane that forms inside the uterus during pregnancy to provide nutrition to the fetus during the pregnancy. It is accomplished by a chemical reaction in the uterus, similar to the cramping that occurs during the female menstrual cycle. God has designed these wave-like motions in the female body that respond to these chemical changes in her uterus. This is why if there is no doctor available and a woman delivers her baby in the desert, the forest, or in a swamp, she can put the baby to her breast immediately after its birth, and it will start the uterus contracting to remove the placenta from the uterus. That is a natural built-in mechanism. These after-birth pains are necessary to release the placenta.

A Cesarean section, *sometimes called C-Section,* is a surgical birth. There are many reasons why a woman may have a Cesarean section. Most C-sections are performed out of a real medical need however; some are planned. For whatever reason you may utilize this method, please know that it is a very critical decision. Keep in mind that this is a major operation and should not be done without serious discussion with your physician.

In most hospitals and birthing centers mothers are often given the drugs Stadol, Fentanyl, or Nubain for pain control. It should be noted that Demerol and Morphine are not commonly used as much as they once were. The anesthetics that are more common in epidurals are Lidocaine (xylocaine), and Bupivicaine (marcaine, marcain). The benefits are obvious in the relief of pain during childbirth. If a mother has been in labor for an extended period of time and is exhausted, an epidural can make the difference between a vaginal birth and a Cesarean section, by allowing her to have some relief so she can sleep and gain new strength. (An epidural is the injection of anesthetic near the spinal cord.) There are, however, some adverse side effects caused by these pain medications. Both you and your baby can experience sleepiness, sedation, dizziness, constipation, sleep problems, insomnia, nausea, vomiting, stomach pain, diarrhea, loss of appetite, memory problems, sweaty, clammy skin, headache, breastfeeding difficulties, bonding difficulties, and withdrawal symptoms. These are the less serious side effects of the pain medications commonly used. Some of the more *serious* adverse effects include: increased need to resuscitate newborns at birth, breathing difficulties in you and your newborn, very rapid heartbeat, very slow heartbeat, confusion, seizures, hallucinations, severe allergic reactions, numbing of face and extremities. These adverse effects are seen in both the mother and the baby.

Most birthing centers do not give these chemicals to their birthing mothers if they are going to breast feed their babies. Often, however, these mothers do not breast feed their babies due to the painful accompanying uterine contractions. Instead most mothers opt for commercially available infant formulas like Infamil/Enfamil. When the mother decides to bypass breast feeding for Infamil/Enfamil, the attending physician administers something to make the uterus contract and they will administer a shot of sintosin /cytosine to dull the pain during the contraction. God engineered breast milk to satisfy the nutritional needs of babies and also to supply immunity to disease through the antibodies from the mother's immune system. It establishes appropriate intestinal flora, which benefits the baby throughout the baby's life. Breastfed babies experience a low incidence of Sudden Infant Death Syndrome, do not suffer from colic, and they more easily excrete dangerous and toxic substances than babies given cow's milk (The People's Doctor, Val. 9, No. 12, P.7).

Physically, you may experience the following:

- **Pain at the episiotomy site.** An e*pisiotomy* is a cut made by your doctor in the *perineum* (the area between the vagina and the anus) to help deliver the baby or prevent tearing. If this was done, or the area was torn during birth, the stitches may make walking or sitting difficult for a period of time. It also can be painful when you cough or sneeze during the healing time.
- **Sore breasts.** Your breasts may be swollen, hard, and painful for several days as your milk comes in. Your nipples may also be sore.
- **Constipation.** As you can imagine having a bowel movement can be difficult for a few days after delivery. Hemorrhoids, episiotomies, and sore muscles can cause pain with bowel movements.
- **Hemorrhoids.** Hemorrhoids (swollen varicose veins in the anal area) are common after pregnancy and delivery.
- **Hot and cold flashes.** Your body's adjustment to changing levels of hormones and blood flow can cause you to perspire one minute and reach for a blanket to cover yourself the next.
- **Urinary or fecal incontinence.** Muscles stretched during delivery, particularly after a long labor, may cause you to leak urine when you laugh or sneeze or may make it difficult to control bowel movements.
- **After pains.** After giving birth, you will continue to experience contractions for a few days as your uterus returns to its pre-pregnancy size. You may notice contractions mostly while your baby is nursing.
- **Vaginal discharge.** *(Lochia).* Immediately following birth you will experience a bloody discharge heavier than a regular

period. Over time, the discharge will fade to white or yellow and then stop entirely within two months.

Emotionally, you may experience irritability, sadness, or crying, commonly referred to as the "baby blues," in the days or weeks after delivery. These symptoms occur in up to 80% of new mothers and may be related to physical changes (including hormone changes and exhaustion) and your emotional adjustment to the responsibilities of caring for a newborn. If these problems persist, inform your doctor or other health professional; you could be experiencing *postpartum depression*. This is a very serious problem that affects between 10% and 25% of new mothers.

You Are A Super Woman! Your Idealistic Dreams of Love, Marriage, Sex, Children and Careers

This is the time of a woman's life journey when she must listen to what her body is telling her. It goes through several cycles each month and if she were to chronicle her feelings as the month goes by, she would notice during the first week a feeling of nesting, meaning that she feels very good emotionally and physically strong. She is ready to tackle the world. (*Here I am world, take me on! As a matter of fact, take your best shot!*) She puts in more hours at work, rises early to exercise and meditate, and volunteers for out-of-town assignments. She is just a body of discipline. This optimistic volt of energy takes place right after the end of her period when her estrogen level is rising. She can take on any project: chairing a committee, baking a cake, cooking a meal, hosting a party or taking the kids on an outing and she never gets tired. She might be coming out of college, starting a career or getting ready to say, "I do."

If this is your season, I charge you to enjoy this one and only life and remember that happiness cannot be traveled to, owned, earned, worn or consumed. Happiness is the spiritual experience of living every minute with love, grace, gratitude, peace, joy, health, and well-being and can only be found inside of you. It exists within just waiting to be discovered. I admonish you not look to the outside world to satisfy your needs and longings. Your outer life only reflects back to you the way you think, feel, and behave. When you search for peace and contentment outside of yourself, you will soon realize what the great Western diseases are-*"I'll be happy when I get more money, . . . when I get a Jaguar, . . . when I get the position I want, etc . . ."* The reality is *"when"* never comes. The only way to find happiness is to understand that happiness is not out there. It is here and it is now. Like beauty, joy is one of the highest vibrations on this planet. God is the highest. Only seeking God will help bring to life the joy that is already inside of you. This special time of life should be enjoyed, for the years go by very fast and the associated changes are rapid.

As a woman's estrogen peaks, others admire her and that only encourages her to do more. Well-being and inner strength ooze from her. Ovulation is occurring. There's a "nesting syndrome." By the third week of a woman's cycle, the same estrogen that gave her that energetic feeling is now being overridden by progesterone. The estrogen high is waning; she is beginning to bleed and irritability kicks in. As the progesterone level rises, she will have good and bad days, emotional ups and downs. This is called PMS. She slows down and most of the time has problems dealing with pressure, people, or even has trouble sleeping. She wants peace and is impatient with her children. She may feel overwhelmed, especially if she is working, or is a leader in her church or community.

Case in Point

I received a telephone call from my friend who is co-pastor of a church with her husband. She was very distraught and angry. She expressed that the people in the church were treating her like a doormat. She was upset that her husband was not speaking up for her. I asked them to come to my office to further discuss the issue. When they came to my office, I asked how things were. She exclaimed while clinging to her husband's arm, "Dr. Morgan, I am fine, I never felt better. I apologize for my demeanor the other day, I don't know what came over me, I was just having a bad day!!" In astonishment, her husband explained that on the day that she called me she was experiencing her monthly PMS symptoms. I could see that he was not comfortable with his wife's affection. He further explained that each month she embarrassed him with loud outbursts at home, at church, or on the street. Then a day or so later, she lavishes him with overwhelming displays of affection. I explained to them that her mood swings were due to the fact that her progesterone levels had lessened, her menstrual cycle was at its end, and her estrogen levels were beginning to peak.

Plan Your Schedule

If a woman gets to know her own body, it is possible for her to manage her schedule in consideration of the vicissitudes of her life. For instance, during the most stressful part of her cycle she can schedule the things that are less stressful. It is imperative that she plans her daily activities around her menstrual cycle. A teacher of young children should not schedule a field trip; nor should an office executive schedule an important meeting during this third week. It will not work.

The fourth week is a better time to handle stressful events or situations. This is when the estrogen in her body is more suitable to dealing with stress. The third week and the days preceding it are called *premenstrual*. This is when the estrogen level falls and many of the emotional and physical symptoms such as crying spells, swollen ankles, social withdrawal, headaches, insomnia (or other sleeping disorders), digestive problems (e.g., diarrhea or constipation), sadness or despair, thoughts of suicide, tension or anxiety, panic attacks, mood swings, lasting irritability or anger, lack of interest in daily activities and relationships, trouble thinking or focusing, tiredness or low energy, food cravings or binge eating, and feeling of out-of-control, etc. will occur. These emotional and physical symptoms are hormonally induced. It is important to remember that not every woman goes through these symptoms; some will have variations of symptoms while others may not have any physical or emotional symptoms at all. These hormone-induced symptoms are not limited to single women in their twenties, but extend to women in general, regardless of whether she is a working professional, blue collar, worker, stay-at-home mom, married or single. A brain chemical called serotonin is said to play a role in *Premenstrual Dysphoric Disorder* (PMDD), a severe form of PMS. It is much more disabling than the normal PMS. In order to be diagnosed with PMDD, she must show signs of five or more of the above symptoms and they must occur during the week before her period and go away after bleeding starts.

Lifestyle Change

Making some lifestyle changes such as those listed below will help to ease some or all of the PMDD symptoms. Traditional treatments with an antidepressant called *selective serotonin reuptake inhibitors* (SSRIs) have been shown to help some women with PMDD. These drugs change serotonin levels in the brain. Serotonin is a neurotransmitter that is involved in the transmission of nerve impulses. Serotonin can trigger the release of substances in the blood vessels of the brain that in turn cause the pain of migraine headaches. Serotonin is also key to mood regulation and pain perception. The following are some of the brands approve by FDA: Sertraline (Zoloft), Fluoxetine (Sarafem), and Paroxetine HCI (Paxil CR). Traditional doctors sometimes recommend birth control pills to treat PMDD. A physician can determine which ones might work best. I do not discount any treatment that meets a woman's needs, however, there are several natural and complementary treatments that work just as well, most without side effects. These natural therapies work much better with natural body radium. Whatever method is chosen, counseling (individual or group), and stress management should be incorporated in this regimen to help relieve symptoms.

Your Gynecological Visit

All women should have an annual Papanicolaou test (also called Pap smear, Pap test, cervical smear, or smear test) beginning at age twenty-one, according to the American College of Obstetricians and Gynecologists. Women 21 to 29 years of age should get a Pap smear every year; then every other year (or as often as your doctor recommends) from ages 30 to 64. It is a screening test to detect potentially pre-cancerous and cancerous cells. To get the most accurate Pap smear results, proper preparation for the annual pelvic exam is required. These simple tips should be followed for more accurate Pap smear results.

What to Avoid Prior to Your Pap Smear:

1. Do not use vaginal douches for at least three days prior to the exam.

2. Refrain from sexual intercourse for forty-eight hours prior to the exam.

3. Do not use tampons, antibiotics, birth control foams or jellies for forty-eight hours prior to the scheduled appointment. These will all cause inflammation.

Tips:

1. Schedule the appointment approximately one or two weeks after you expect your period. If your period starts, call your provider to reschedule.

2. Write down any questions you have for your doctor, and take your list to your appointment.

3. Don't forget to inform your doctor about any infections, discharges, or pain you have experienced since your last examination. If you have had previous abnormal Pap smear results that your physician may not have on record, let them know about them. Also be certain to tell them if you know you've been exposed to HPV.

4. If you receive abnormal results, get a detailed explanation about the meaning from your provider. If you don't understand, ask questions.

5. Follow your physician's advice about any further diagnostic/treatment procedures. Remember, too, that it's always your right to ask for a second opinion.

Pap Smear Classifications:

Class 1-The results are fine.
Class 1-The physician may have some concerns; there may be some inflammation or bacteria in the area.
Class 3-There may be evidence of advanced inflammation and or bacteria in the area.
Class 4 & 5-There may be some suspicion of cancer cells in the area.

Twelve Things Every Woman in Her Twenties Should Know

Being in my twenties is what I waited for all my life. I realize it is a crucial period in my life. It's my transitional time when I should be discovering my true self and when I really became a woman. I realize it's an awesome time! I graduated from college two years ago. Today I am leaving home to live on my own. I started my career last year, and am building new relationships while learning what it really means to grow up. Between bills, and my early morning wake ups, it's easy to lose sight of the fun side of life. That being said, do you have any advice for me as I go through this season of life? Thank you, Joy

Here are twelve nuggets to ensure you maximize these once-in-a-lifetime opportunities that will never come your way again. Treasure, learn, and enjoy every moment during these special years:

1. **No subtitles.** One of the mistakes I made when I was in my twenties was connecting my happiness to external factors. It is easy to use things such as your relationships, friends, looks, and money to determine just how happy you are and how happy you will become. When things are going great, external things make you feel fantastic. The problem occurs when things are going bad and you are having a rough time. In this case it only makes us feel terrible. According to the universal law of attraction, we only get more of the things that we are focusing on. If things are going bad in our life right now and we focus on it that means we will only get more bad things happening to us in the future. If you have ever been in love you understand how wonderful of a feeling it is. You feel like you are walking on air and everything seems to go your way. Everything is brighter and there are tons of possibilities for your future. Why not learn to fall in love with your life in general? Why not get that same feeling every time you get up and think about the world in which you live?

2. **Learn how to manage your budget**. Most women start taking care of their own finances at this age. Learning how to manage a budget for rent, groceries, utilities, while also setting aside a little "fun or mad money" and a little savings can be difficult. I've found that tracking your monthly income and all your ancillary costs can help you better understand what you're spending so you know what you're able to save. There are actually several apps to help you keep track of that. (e.g., Mint.com) This is also a time to think ahead and start your 401K. If you work for a company that offers this type of plan, be sure to ask your Human Resources Department to help you set it up.

3. **Cherish your friendships**. These years are usually filled with a lot of dating, a lot of love, along with a lot of time mending broken hearts. It's important to realize that guys will come and go, but a solid group of friends will be there to help you through it all forever. Even when you do find the one you'll spend the rest of your life with; remember that your friends

will be the support system you need through the good and the bad. The lesson here—Don't forego important friendships in lieu of a relationship. Create balance. Good friends are hard to find.

4. **Dress to impress**. At this point in your life, you have fully grown into your beautiful body, which means there are no more excuses for trying to squeeze into that mini skirt you wore during your senior year of high school. It's time to accept your body and all of its beautifully unique assets by dressing accordingly. Your twenties is a time to experiment and learn what works best for your body type. Find out what kind of jeans are the right fit for your figure, what size dress is most appropriate for your shape, and embrace what you are working with. Accepting your shape will help you look and feel your best. Confidence is key for any twenty-something who is about to take on the world.

5. **Don't make the same mistake twice**. People often say that your twenties is the time to make mistakes. But what's important about this is not the act of actually making the mistake itself, but rather *learning* from the lessons these mistakes teach us. Whether it's a slip-up in a relationship or at your job, don't get down on yourself that it happened. Instead, take it as a lesson learned and promise yourself it won't happen again. *"If I ran a school, I'd give the average grade to the ones who gave me all the right answers, for being good parrots. I'd give the top grades to those who made a lot of mistakes and told me about them, and then told me what they learned from them."*—R. Buckminster Fuller

6. **Speak up for yourself**. As you begin to take on your independence in your twenties, it's important to learn when to stand up for yourself. Get yourself the raise you deserve, tell your friends when they are treating you poorly, let that barista at Starbucks know that she gave you the wrong drink. If you never say anything, nothing will ever change, and those negative things will build up. Remember that you're a strong,

beautiful and independent woman, and speaking up for yourself is important in leading the life you desire.

7. **Know how to take a compliment**. Confidence is the key to taking on the world as a twenty-something. Part of that confidence is knowing how to accept a compliment. When someone tells you you're beautiful, accept it and say *thank you* (and maybe even blush a little). Accepting a compliment unveils your confidence and comfort in your own skin, which is an attractive quality for all women. That kind of self-assuredness can help you do anything from landing you the perfect job to meeting the man of your dreams.

8. **You don't always have to be right**. With the confidence that comes in your twenties, sometimes it's hard to know when to set your stubbornness aside. It takes a lot of biting your tongue to learn this lesson, however, *you don't always have to be right*! You will come across situations where it's incredibly hard to do, particularly when you know you're right. But sometimes it's best to save your relationship with that person (especially if it's in the work place) than to hold the upper hand. Your twenties is a time to learn when it's okay to stand up for yourself, but also understand the moments when you just need to back away.

9. **Don't lose the child within**. I have to say, out of all of these points, the number one thing to remember is to *never lose sight of yourself*. You grow up a lot in your twenties, but you're still young enough to have fun and bring out the little girl that's still left in you. You'll have plenty of time to continue to grow up, settle down, have children, and worry about spending too much money. But your twenties is only a stepping-stone to that point. So go have a crazy night out with your girlfriends, get set up on a blind date, buy that expensive pair of shoes you can't really afford, be weird and goofy, and go on adventures! These are the memories you'll cherish when you look back on these years.

10. **Eat well.** Now's the time to take charge of your health, the healthy things you choose today will pay off with interest in the future. Eating better is a good place to start. Choose whole-grain foods, deep-colored fruits and vegetables, and lower-fat dairy products. When you eat your meals, include a couple of servings of fish per week. Go easy on red meat and foods that are high in fat, sugar, or salt. Limit intake of caffeine, alcohol, and spicy foods, which may contribute to high blood pressure and diabetes. Do a natural cleanse or detox every three months and please see your health care professional yearly.

11. **Manifest your thoughts**. Learn to manifest your desires, it will help you bring your desires into reality so that you're living the joyous and fulfilling life you deserve. Desires such as relationships, health issues, finances, career concerns, and more are influenced by this law that governs your time/space reality and you'll discover powerful processes that will help you go with the positive flow of life. It's your birthright to live a life filled with everything that is good and this book will show you how to make it so in every way! *A dear friend of mine had been working very actively on manifesting her dreams. She created a bucket list and vision board for what she wanted in her life. Some were small, like buying a bike, and others were on a grander scale for family, marriage and community. She even wrote a check to herself from God for an outlandish amount she thought she deserved. One day she said to me, "I have a weird confession to make to you. I wrote a check from God to me for $1,530,450. What do you think?" I gave her a verse, "For as a man thinks in his heart, so is he"-Proverbs 23:7. Less than two weeks after making vision boards and writing her check, her father whom she did not know, suddenly passed away. She was notified that she and her sister both were to receive a sizeable amount of money from a Swiss bank account she never knew about. Turns out it was for the exact amount she wrote on her vision check.*

12. **Put your trust in God.** This should have been number one, however, when a man or woman has faith, all the mountains of the world cannot turn them back. Yes, with faith you will endure any trial, any disaster, and nothing will weaken you. But one who is not a true believer, one who lacks real faith, will lament over the least disappointment, and cry out against the slightest thing that mars their peace and pleasure. Never lose your trust in God. *"Be thou ever hopeful, for the bounties of God will never cease to flow upon you." Ruhi.* Through all your conditions immerse yourself in the sea of God's blessings and He thoroughly will direct your path. When you put your whole trust and confidence in Him who created you he will be with you through your life journey. *"Trust in the LORD with all thine heart; and lean not unto thine own understanding. In all thy ways acknowledge him, and he shall direct thy paths."* (Proverbs 3: 5-6)

The Super-Woman's Nutritional Needs

Natural Treatments

Women in their twenties lead active lives and need adequate nutrition to support their minds and bodies. Nutritional gaps can occur if a young woman is not eating a balanced diet. While supplements are not designed to take the place of whole foods, a multivitamin can help fill in gaps that cannot be met through diet alone. Your individual needs may vary greatly so consulting a competent physician regarding your nutritional requirement (vitamin, mineral, amino acids, etc., supplementation) is recommended.

Calcium:

Studies suggest that calcium levels are lower in women with PMS and that calcium supplementation reduces the severity of symptoms. A large study looked at 1,057 women with PMS and 1,968 women without PMS. Women with the greatest intake of calcium from food sources had the least PMS symptoms. 300 mg of calcium carbonate four times a day significantly reduced bloating, depression, pain, mood swings, and food cravings.

Chaste Tree Berry

Chaste tree berry (*Vitex agnus-castus*) is one of the most popular herbs for premenstrual syndrome in Europe. A study published in the *British Medical Journal* involving 178 women with PMS found that chaste tree berry significantly reduced PMS symptoms over three menstrual cycles. Women taking chaste tree berry had significant improvements in irritability, depression, headaches, and breast tenderness. The most common side effects of chaste tree berry are nausea, headache, digestive disturbances, menstrual disorders, acne, itching, and skin rashes. Chaste tree berry should not be taken by pregnant or nursing women. The safety of chaste tree berry in children or people with kidney or liver disease has not been established. Theoretically, chaste tree berry may interact with hormones or drugs that affect the pituitary gland.

Magnesium

The mineral magnesium, found naturally in food and available in supplements, has shown good preliminary results for PMS. One study examined the use of magnesium supplements or a placebo in thirty-two women with PMS. The amount of magnesium used was 360 mg three times a day, starting from day 15 to the start of the menstrual period. Magnesium supplements were found to significantly improve PMS mood changes.

Evening Primrose Oil

Evening Primrose Oil is a plant oil that contains gamma-linolenic acid, an omega-6 essential fatty acid. Gamma-linolenic acid is involved in the metabolism of hormone-like substances called *prostaglandins* that regulate pain and inflammation in the body.

Acupuncture

The liver is the organ most affected by stress, anger, frustration, stagnation energy ("qi"), emotions, alcohol, and spicy and fatty foods that can lead to PMS symptoms such as breast tenderness, abdominal bloating, and cramping. Acupuncture, a traditional Chinese medicine, along with exercise, expressing emotions, and breathing exercises are recommended by practitioners to relieve liver stagnation.

Dietary Suggestions

- Reduce sugar and salt intake. This is especially useful for bloating and swelling of the hands and feet, breast tenderness, and dizziness. Increase foods rich in potassium, such as fish, beans, and broccoli.
- Eat small, frequent meals to help stabilize blood sugar.
- Eliminate caffeine, which can aggravate anxiety, depression, and breast tenderness.
- Increase intake of fruits, vegetables, beans, nuts, seeds, and fish.
- Avoid alcohol.
- Decrease intake of fatty foods and red meat.

Exercise

Regular aerobic exercise such as brisk walking, jogging, swimming, or cycling may help relieve PMS symptoms. In one study, the frequency but not the intensity of exercise was associated with decreased PMS symptoms.

Relaxation

Breathing exercises, meditation, aromatherapy, and yoga are some natural ways to reduce stress and promote relaxation. Many women feel more assertive and attuned to their needs in the weeks before menses. This can be used constructively by allowing for personal time to relax, expressing emotions, and giving priority to your needs and what nourishes you.

Other Natural Remedies for PMS:

- Ginkgo
- Vitamin E
- Royal jelly
- OPCs (oligomeric proanthocyanidins)
- Uva ursi
- St. John's wort
- Wild yam
- Dandelion
- Reflexology
- Chiropractic medicine
- Massage therapy
- Progesterone cream

Your Spiritual Needs

It is most important that you seek to become attached to your source. The plant must remain attached to the soil for food, the fish to the water, and you to your Creator. Anytime you are not connected to your source, your spiritual life suffers. To be spiritual has nothing to do with religion. In my personal journey, I have met many religious people who are not spiritual people. Your spiritual life includes your spiritual practices such as prayer, meditation, and the path it will take for you to get closer to your God. It also includes your interactions with your community and other human beings. Here are some steps you can take to improve your spiritual life.

Step 1: Grow and develop

Spiritual growth and development is a process that needs to be cultivated every minute of your life. Unlike skills you may have, your spiritual life is your life force and without it life would be chaotic. To cultivate a healthy spiritual life, pray, meditate, and gather with other like-minded people. Do whatever it takes in order to be lined up with your spiritual belief. For example, if you are a Christian, read your Bible, pray, attend church, give, and increase your knowledge of God through accepting Jesus Christ. If you are a Buddhist, that list would look quite different toward your journey to spirituality. The holy life in Buddhism begins and ends in practice, not belief and doctrine.

Step 2: Forgive and give thanks

I believe that forgiving another person is an act of liberation. It frees you both from the negativity that exists between you and that person, and it frees you from holding a grudge and the negative emotions that come with it. You should also express your gratitude, or count your blessings for your family, friends, neighbors and even everyday things like your finances, home, car or pet. To be thankful for all that you have and to express that gratitude will enhance your spiritual growth and better your spiritual life.

Step 3: Seek spiritual help where necessary along the way

There are numerous outlets that offer spiritual and other help: Church, a pastor, a rabbi, a therapist, a friend, or family members. You can seek help through prayer. Prayer is the act of actively seeking contact with God. Prayer may be used in countless ways to encourage peace, wisdom, healing, and spiritual guidance. You can seek spiritual help at churches to assist you in growing in your faith. If you're seeking spiritual growth, don't be afraid to ask for guidance.

Apart from God, talking about your thoughts and feelings with a supportive person can also make you feel better. It can be very healing, in and of itself, to voice your worries or talk about something that's weighing on your mind. And it feels good to be listened to, and to know that someone else cares about you and wants to help.

It can even be very helpful to talk about your problems to close friends and family members. But sometimes, we need help that the people around us aren't qualified or able to provide. When you need extra support, an outside perspective, or some expert guidance, talking to a therapist or counselor can be very helpful. While the support of friends and family is important, therapy is different. Therapists are professionally-trained listeners who can help you get to the root of your problems, overcome emotional challenges, and make positive changes in your life.

Step 4: Mature in your spirituality
Although you may not realize it, it is essential to invest in and develop all aspects of your personal life of which your spirituality is the most important component. When you develop spiritually, you, as a human being are much closer to achieving the feeling of completeness necessary for total fulfillment than any other living creature. I am not talking about church, but your relationship with God and your fellow mankind. In my opinion, the depth of spirituality defines your character. When we are spiritual, our character traits exemplify goodness. We have the ability to rise above our materialistic, worldly existence, and make the connection with the highest power of our universe, who I call God!

The Four Spiritual Components of Women

- Your Physical Body, Your Intellect, Your Spirit, and Your Soul.
- Spirituality encompasses the spirit and the soul. The *Soul* is manifested through your consciousness—emotions, thoughts, will, desire, conscience, affection, intuition, perception, and self-awareness.
- The *Spirit* is manifested by our character—temperament, disposition, tendency, individuality, habits, frame of mind, ambition and drive.

Spiritual fullness or fulfillment can give a woman the kind of wisdom that, when put into practice, can enhance her life in unimaginable ways. In the process of making the spiritual connection, she will discover a level of awareness necessary to cleanse her spirit and purify her soul. As she matures spiritually, she will begin to flourish in ways she only dreamed of. Only when her spiritual life is healthy can a positive transformation begin to take place in her life. I realize at this stage of life most women only see positive things ahead, however, it is important that she does not forget the source of her power. Our natural tendency as human beings is to continue to develop as we move toward achieving only goodness in our life. By feeding our souls with spiritual food, we are better positioned to make the positive changes we desire.

Our spiritual life serves as a compass or GPS. When the storms of life become difficult, we can receive spiritual guidance and direction. It will help in attaining clarity that will eliminate all the negatives that can devour your journey. It has been said, "We are not human beings on a spiritual journey; we are spiritual beings on a human journey." Even with this knowledge, we have become a society with a culture that places great emphasis on acquiring external things, amassing wealth, fame, and material possessions. Because of this, it is easy to lose the focus on the internal self and the higher consciousness needed to nurture our spirit. It is the spirit that feeds the soul and produces the essence of who we are. Affiliating with a particular religion does not guarantee a pure spirit, because sometimes religion can be the biggest hindrance. It takes a conscious effort to purify the soul and cleanse the spirit. When a woman's spirit is cleansed she will display characteristics of spiritual wellness, love, compassion, joy, happiness, peace, kindness, tolerance, faith, humility, self-control, motivation, determination, ambition, gratitude, honesty, and forgiveness.

Spiritual maturity is learning to live and love like Jesus did, rather than in a human way. It is choosing to live in a God-like manner in everyday situations. To be spiritually mature is to love God with all your heart and all your soul, and to love your neighbor as you love yourself. Spiritual growth is an ongoing process, with a goal of being one with God.

Remember your twenties are years of change. He has carefully crafted you with an individual destiny. Graceful aging is more about a woman's character than her figure or looks. The sort of daughter our Heavenly Father desires is found in 1 Peter 3:3-4: "*Whose adorning let it not be that outward adorning of plaiting the hair, and of wearing of gold, or of putting on of apparel; But let it be the hidden man of the heart, in that which is not corruptible, even the ornament of a meek and quiet spirit, which is in the sight of God of great price."*

What makes a woman beautiful? Her Heavenly Father beautifies her, as He has shaped her self-image and given her talents and confidence to change the world for Him. The older a woman gets, the more beautiful she should become, because true beauty is inward, a heart connecting with God.

What makes a woman beautiful? Her Heavenly Father beautifies her, as He has shaped her self-image and God's women, His queens, His princesses, and His special daughters are connected to Him. Whatever her age, He still sees her as a child. A woman's personal relationship with her Heavenly Father affects her beauty, heart, health, and character. In the Old Testament of the Biblical text, God gave Sarah, Rebekah, and Esther outward beauty. But these women also loved God. Be aware that no measure of physical attractiveness can compensate for the inner beauty of the heart that seeks God. I have met many women who lived their lives without a relationship with God and bitterness, deceit, and hardness of heart is often evident. Going to a church doesn't change that fact, but a mature lady who has been filled with the Spirit of God is radiant. She is contented. Her heart is soft and full of His love. For years, her Heavenly Father has been gently influencing her soul. It is not too late to start becoming a Spiritual woman. Your health may be uncertain and genetics can play a part in the ailment you suffer, but God still has your back. The Bible promises: "Be not be wise in thine own eyes: fear the LORD and depart from evil. It shall be health to thy navel, and marrow to thy bones." (Provers 3:7-8). Give your body, mind and emotions to Him, for He cares for you.

> Proverbs 31 speaks of the wife of noble character. "Be not deceived: evil communications corrupt good manners." (1 Corinthians 15:33) Your twenties and thirties make up a decade of potential character growth and deepened faith. God's blueprint for your life is

perfect. He knows how to tie all your goals together, and He will accomplish His dreams for your life.

You need to be intentional about your days, living them with Godly purpose and contentment. Daily disciplines will cultivate a heart that pleases God. Whether you travel as a single woman, experiencing different cultures, or you become a wife and mother during these years of change, God's awesome creation will inspire you. And God wants you to look to Him for help to be that beautiful lady He created you to be. You will become a woman of poise, grace, godliness, and purpose.

A wonderful woman

- Your strengths are amazing
- You can handle trouble
- And carry heavy burdens

A wonderful woman

- Holds happiness, love and opinions

A wonderful woman

- Smiles when you feel like screaming
- Sings when you feel like crying
- Cries when you are happy
- And laughs when you are afraid

A wonderful woman

- Your love is unconditional
- But there is one thing wrong with you,
- You sometimes forget what you are worth
- That's my wonderful woman.

-Bibi. W. Kaudur

Recommended Books for Childbearing Woman

I would like to recommend reading *Wise Woman Herbal for the Childbearing Years* by Susun S. Weed and Janice Novet. I found this book to be informative and simple, a plus for any woman especially those of childbearing age. The authors address herbs that are helpful for pregnancy, childbirth, lactation, and newborns, etc.

Ms. Weed and Ms. Novet share several formulas that are recommended for all women however, their suggested formulas has been put together for women during their childbearing years. These formulas are confirmed favorites with pregnant women, midwives, childbirth educators, and new parents. Women who use these formulas start taking them two months before their pregnancy. Most of the women I spoke to who use these formulas found them to be effective for birth control, or to help ensure pregnancy, even in the most difficult of situations.

Chapter Six

STAGE THREE-MIDLIFE MALAISE: THE EMOTIONAL WATERSHED (AGES 35-45)

It's been a long journey toward this biological milestone of premenopause, but your body has been preparing for this for a lifetime. This time the changes will be a bit different and can be daunting and unsettling if you are not prepared or do not understand why they are happening.

You have seen some hormonal and metabolic changes in the past decade that have resulted in a different body shape: your waist looks less pronounced, your breasts seem less firm, your hips and thighs are more rounded and more generous than in the past. You think you are gaining weight and try to battle against your changing shape by vigorously exercising and dieting, but you find that eating less doesn't work as a defense mechanism against hormonal body changes. As a matter of fact any changes in diet may exaggerate your hormones.

When my "queen" was in her twenties, each month her stomach would get puffy before her period, but after her period all the bloating would go away. In her mid-thirties, her stomach began to look as if she were bloated all the time (and mine too!) I have noticed the same thing with many of my female clients and friends in that age range. They often say, "Look at my stomach, do you think I need a colonic?"

Many of the female clients that have visited my office have been on numerous diets, fads, detoxifications, and fasting programs, since I met them, without any significant changes in their body shape. Most of them felt their hips and thighs were larger, and their pants were no longer comfortable. Many of them didn't know what was going on and inquired about very low calorie diets.

What most of these women did not understand was that their bodies were responding to changes not only in their hormone levels but in their metabolic rates. Researchers do not fully understand why the rate at which the body converts food to energy slows down as we age, but it may in fact be part of an intricate relationship between the hormones that govern a host of reproductive and metabolic functions. Aside from the metabolic changes, the body is also changing the way it produces estrogen. When you were younger, your ovaries were the primary manufacturing sites for two types of estrogen, *estradiol* and *estrone*. During perimenopause, as women's ovaries age and produce less of both of these types of estrogen, nature assigns estrone synthesis to her fat cells. Eventually her ovaries stop producing estrogen completely.

During the perimenopausal years, your fat cells assume this important function that your ovaries once performed. In fact, it is healthy for you to have enough fat cells to create the estrone your body requires. As you journey to the next stage of life, your body will store more fat cells in your upper arms, abdomen, buttocks, and thighs. So that rounded, softer or sometimes spongy look you now have or will acquire is actually the look of health and a sign of nature's protection for your body.

Some women at midlife exhibit few if any perimenopausal symptoms—no loss of libido, no hot flashes, no vaginal dryness, no depression, and no mood swings. In fact, the only changes they may observe are shorter menstrual cycles, lighter periods, and a little weight gain around their waist and breasts. This, however, is not the norm.

Although it is normal and healthy for women to develop softer and rounder figures as their ovarian function declines, excessive weight is not healthy. Being seriously overweight elevates the risk of heart disease, lymphatic disease, and other illnesses. As a college student, I had many posters of my favorite female entertainers and models. They were all thin with very few fat cells on their bodies. Fifteen to twenty years later, most of their lean bodies had changed into what I would call "positively plump" bodies. Midlife realities had caught up with them. I have not met very many women in their late thirties and forties who look the same as they did in their twenties. It was the baby boom generation that gave rise to the current idea that woman must be thin. While women of this age now are taking a lead in dismantling this notion, there are still very strong media messages that slim is elegant, rich, and disciplined while other body shapes are sloppy and lacking in class, or even intelligence.

The Watershed Observations of Discontent

One of my clients, Dora, was always on a diet or in the gym. She came to my office because she felt none of the diets were giving her the desired results she wanted. Her kitchen cabinets were filled with pills, potions, powders, and drinks, none of which seemed to work to give her the body she desired. I looked at her and saw that she had a beautiful body, was not overweight, bloated, or in pain; her body was firm and in tremendous condition. She was dismayed, however, because of the hormonally induced changes in her body, specifically her upper arms, abdomen, buttocks, and thighs. She felt fine and had no physical problems except her perception of how others viewed her. She had invested a lot of her money and time in maintaining her body image and she was not getting the desired results. She told us of her surgeries, actually four tucks, one each to her upper arms, abdomen, and thighs. She was not happy with the results and believed she was left disfigured. Dora wanted a quick fix to her situation and was not receptive to any treatment that did not bring her immediate gratification. The Bible states, "My people are destroyed for lack of knowledge: . . ." (Hosea 4:6 KJV). If Dora had allowed me to explain why her body was changing rapidly before her eyes, she would not been in that irreversible predicament. I suggested she speak to a therapist, something she emphatically said she would not do. At our last meeting she said she thinking of undergoing corrective surgery although I advised her that it would not produce the results she desired. Her final word was, "I don't care how much I have to spend, I'm going to look the way I did two years ago."

Observation

What a wonderful opportunity it would have been for Dora to turn this perception of body image around. She could have replaced the goal of an idealized body shape with the conviction that her body was changing in the way nature intended and that her goal should be fitness, strength, and tone rather than slim. Sometimes surgery can enhance a person's self-image. It will not correct a defect in personality, but can bring out a hidden facet of your personality.

The Watershed Observations Of Discontent Continues

To look at her I would describe her as breathtaking, enigmatic, sweet, incredible, spunky, upbeat, friendly, riveting, exhilarating, well dressed and even smart-looking. She was a 35-year-old pharmacology graduate and Brooklyn, New York native. She had a scheduled appointment for a job interview. Her résumé said she was a graduate of Columbia University with an MSc in Clinical Pharmacology. I was very impressed with her résumé as were my colleagues. As the interview commenced, the personality she revealed was a total contradiction to her physical image or the one portrayed by her résumé. When we asked her to tell us a little about herself, Ms. Carter forgot that she was having a job interview and instead had an emotional flashback of her college years and how her deadbeat, womanizing father abandoned her mother and her for another woman, and how her mother refused to help her with her tuition. Because of the rage and anger that came out of her, we stopped the interview. Ms. Carter called a few days later to inquire whether she had been chosen for the position. I told her we had chosen someone else. Again she had a tantrum, but this time it was directed towards me. Two years later while at a neighborhood shopping center, I ran into Ms. Carter, who was working in the pharmacy. She recognized me and again blamed me for her not giving her the position she wanted. Her supervisor overheard the exchange and came over to apologize to me for her behavior. He said he was considering letting her go because of her frequent outbursts of rage. I was able to convince her supervisor to give her another chance. I then begged Ms. Carter to give me another chance as well. It took a month of my asking and gaining her trust before she consented. When she came to my office for an evaluation, I found that Ms. Carter's hormones were imbalanced. After an initial body de-tox, followed by one month on a hormonal protocol, she became the lovely person that first stood before me at her job interview.

A Follow-up Letter From Ms. Carter

Three years ago I remember waking up with symptoms of menopause. I was thirty-seven years of age, just graduating with my Masters Degree in pharmacology. I did not realize it was menopause; I did know something was wrong with me. At the time I thought I was going crazy, [with] crazy mood swings. I would get upset and angry at a drop of a hat. I blamed everybody and anybody for every and anything at any time. I had problems sleeping at night. It was almost unbearable; I would sweat all night. During the day I would be exhausted. During that time I went to seven different doctors and specialists. All said I was too young to be going through menopause, and if it were menopause I would have weight gain. I was given several tests for menopause including FSH (follicle stimulating hormones) and LH (luteinizing hormones). Both FSH and LH levels came back low indicating I was not in perimenopause or menopause, which meant I had some other medical issue. But my doctors kept saying my symptoms were in my head. It is now one year after starting my hormone regulation protocol and I can't believe how wonderful I feel. Most of my friends are back in my life. I am still trying to mend my relationship with my parents. Dr. Morgan recommended me for a research position at a large pharmaceutical company. I love my new position and my

100

renewed life. Thank you, Dr. Morgan, I owe my life to you and I recommend your wisdom to all women regardless of their age.

Thank you and God bless you,
M. Carter MSc

Some of the women who experience hormone imbalance range from nineteen to sixty years of age. I would recommend a full medical examination by a competent physician be done before commencing on any of these therapies.

Keep in mind, to resolve hormonal imbalance, you should look at more than estrogen. That's not the case with some conventional practitioners who seem to want to focus solely on estrogen levels. While your estrogen levels are important, so are progesterone and testosterone levels, as well as their ratios to each other, as well as to insulin, cortisol and thyroid levels. For example, your estrogen levels may appear high, when in reality, they are holding steady while your progesterone levels are dropping.

I also advise women to look at all the areas of their lives and imagine each of the areas as if they were four bank accounts: One account for relationships with others; the second account for what they have achieved, the third for their physical appearance, and the fourth account is their relationship with God. Next, think of the emphasis, time, attention, effort, and energy expended in these areas in terms of money and observe where most of the "money" is deposited. If all of the money is in the bank account labeled "body image," you will be disappointed as your body begins to change.

If a woman is now in her forties and her breasts are still upright, firm, and pointing like torpedoes, they are either very blessed or their breasts are made of silicone (especially if they have had children). When a woman has children her breasts lose quite a bit of the fatty tissue and muscle mass. Unless she exercises regularly, her breasts will quickly lose their muscle tone. Aerobic exercise is great for the cardiovascular system but it does very little to build muscles. Only weight-bearing exercises build muscle. We all remember Jane Fonda and others who exercised and got their bodies to eye candy status in their forties and fifties, but in their sixties they became slaves to Botox and laser treatments.

The Midlife Slump

The Midlife Woman. These three words are capable of striking fear in the hearts of many 35 to 45 year old women. Keep in mind that both men and women go through stages or cycles in their lives, and progress naturally from infancy to childhood to adulthood. Each cycle helps us to build on the previous cycle. Parts of ourselves die with each cycle and are transformed in order that we may move into the next stage, leaving only memories. Each stage is usually welcomed with anticipation and excitement. When women reach midlife, the excitement and anticipation may come to an abrupt end. Society (and therefore women) have viewed this period of a woman's life as a potential downward spiral of fading productivity, usefulness, influence, power, and beauty. Physical beauty is often defined as youthfulness, slenderness, naiveté, and innocence. Our society is prejudiced against aging in general, and doubles that prejudice toward the idea that a middle-aged or mature woman is a vital, beautiful, powerful trustee of our society. Middle age makes women miserable, so they should not blame their job, kids, spouse, income (or lack of it). It is time to understand why these changes and moods are taking place.

From Denial to Transformation

Most of the women I know feel that this stage of life is a doorway to an empty life: once they go through it life is over, but there is life after the midlife stump.

Before menopause, there is a stage called perimenopause. *Perimenopause,* the period leading up to *menopause,* can be difficult for women at first. Some women wonder if their body will be able to withstand the barrage of problems that come with menopause.

Others see it as the "beginning of the end" and still others feel it is a time to enjoy life.

Remember, menopause is not a single moment in time; it can represent thirty years of life or more in our youth-obsessed culture. Be advised, anything short of optimal health and balance for any woman does not have to be tolerated. One woman told me she was in denial that she was indeed going through *perimenopause*. She was in denial for years before finding relief for her physical issues and, ultimately, peace of mind about her place in the world. Wherever a woman may be on her journey through perimenopause, the symptoms she feels ultimately influence her actions and reactions. Women, you must know that you do have the power to help yourselves during this time. For many of you, it will be a wonderful time of growth and transformation.

Time Of Reflection And Questioning Of Life Choices

The transition between young and old can happen in a blink of an eye. It can begin the moment one buries his or her last parent, or notices an age spot, or becomes the head of the family. How did this happen? Or it can begin the moment a woman catches her reflection in a shop window and does a double take because the image she sees resembles her mother. The moment of realization that youth has vanished and that midlife is now a reality, is what the French call becoming "a woman of a certain age." It is a moment that can propel a woman into years of reflection and self-examination: *"What have I done with my life so far?" "Where am I going?" "What am I going to do with the rest of my life?"* It is also a moment that can and should launch her into an energizing time of self-discovery and personal growth.

When does this time of reflection and questioning start? Well, for some women, developing a sense of their own aging and starting the transition from youth into middle age happens in their thirties. Some begin in their forties, and others as late as their fifties. Again, this depends on the emotional and physical foundation set in place years earlier. I remember several of my female clients in their mid-thirties or forties saying to me, "I looked in the mirror and saw wrinkles. What can I do to get rid of them?" When I looked at their faces I did not see any wrinkles. To these women, however, the reality of the reflection looking back at them from the mirror was a sign that they were losing their youth. I started this book with the premise of a single word "CHANGE!" Checking the mirror for wrinkles, looking for sags, and investigating skin tone are not what you bargained for but you know it will happen one day.

Case in Point

A woman I met named Barbara comes to mind. She was tall, slender, with a short afro hair style and the most beautiful, soul-searching brown eyes. She was concerned with the environment, the fate of her soul, and the trajectory of her career. She was intelligent and well-respected by her superiors and colleagues at the law firm where she was employed, but being sexy was never her priority. Yet, even Barbara was not happy with the physical changes she saw happening to her thirty-eight year old body. She was not concerned about her graying hair, which she described as looking "frosted." She was concerned with the crinkles at the corners of her eyes, the bags under her eyes, her new tendency to gain weight. I tried to be philosophical with Barbara but it did not work. She said candidly, "I caught a little glimpse of myself in a shop window as I walked down the street and thought to myself, "When did that happen?" "When did it happen?" I asked her.

"I wish I could tell you that. I looked into the mirror one day and saw suddenly the cruelest fact of life: I was old. But the truth was sadder than that. My mirror until that day was a faithful friend. That day for the first time, I noticed I was thirty-eight. I knew how old I was but never noticed it. Two attractive men chatted disinterestedly to each other, so I did what I had always done, strutted foxily (I thought) to join them; only to be politely, but obviously, rebuffed. A nearby friend rescued me with a glass of wine and a whisper: "Not as easy as it used to be, is it?""

How Did I Get Here?

"I am thirty-one, I saw on television today that by the age of twenty-eight, most women believe they have started to lose their looks. By thirty-one, most think they have passed their prime. Alright, I don't believe that is strictly true, but I would love to look the way I did when I was eighteen. I have a photograph of me taken at the age 20, when I was backpacking around Europe after my second year in college. Even though I haven't looked at it for years, I can describe it in minute detail. After weeks in the sun, I was beautifully bronzed. My glossy hair cascaded in perfect chestnut curls, (grey hairs had yet to be invented), my skin was clear (post teen spots, pre fine lines) and my stomach concaved naturally rather than the result of hours in a gym). To me, that photo sums up my glorious youth. And part of me believes that my skin has never been so radiant, my hair so lustrous and my body so toned since.

Of course, at the time I didn't think I'd reached my beauty nirvana and that it would be all downhill from then on in. No, I think I was at least, oh, twenty-six, when that happened. I remember doing my make-up in the mirror and catching sight of a fleck of silver. Realizing, with what can only be described as horror, that it was a grey hair, I gasped audibly, plucked it out and phoned my best friend to announce in melodramatic fashion, 'Oh my god, I'm getting old!' With all the drama queenery of my proclamation, there was some truth behind it. Wrinkles and grey hair to me spelled old. That single grey hair was proof that I had begun my journey down the slippery slope. Yes, of course, in my heart of hearts I knew that there is a beauty to be found in age, wisdom, and self-confidence. It's just like many of the women who think at age thirty one, they've lost their looks, I'm just not entirely sure I'd choose that sort of beauty over the beauty that lies in being eighteen.—Bev in Brooklyn

Observation

Unfortunately, many women feel like Beverly. Dr. Gergen explains that the "the cultural imperative that how we look determines how valuable we are to ourselves, our men, our world is what makes women so inordinately sensitive to the physical signs of aging." Still?

Yes, still. Despite the fact that they hold positions such as Secretary of State, judges, professors, and executives. Psychologists have found that most women still think that how they look rather than what they do is what gives them value.

I Would Like To Get Pregnant

"I just turned thirty-seven and am now ready to have a child, but I am wondering just how hard it's going to be to get pregnant. My husband is thirty-nine. What can we do to up our chances?

Be blessed,
Sam

Many women today find themselves trying to conceive after the age of thirty-five. This opportunity can be full of joys and riddled with new questions. Despite the challenges, many women in their thirties and forties successfully conceive. The most common cause of age-related decline in fertility is less frequent ovulation. As women age, they begin to have occasional cycles where an egg is never released. Egg quality and quantity also declines in a woman's thirties and forties. Other reasons conceiving after thirty-five may be more difficult include:

- Infection or surgery that caused scar tissue around the fallopian tubes or cervix
- Endometriosis
- Fibroids or uterine disorders
- Decrease in cervical fluid
- Chronic health problems such as high blood pressure or diabetes

Miscarriage is also more common in women over thirty-five. This is often caused by the increased incidence of chromosomal abnormalities. Women age 35 to 45 have a 20-35 % chance of miscarriage. Trying to conceive after thirty-five may seem overwhelming, but there are many things that can be done to make getting pregnant easier. Here are some things to remember:

- Schedule a pre-conception appointment with your health practitioner. You and your health care provider can review your medical history, current medications, and overall lifestyle. This gives you the opportunity to address any concerns about trying to conceive after age thirty-five. After age thirty-five women who is physically, mentally, and emotionally healthy is more likely to conceive and be healthy throughout her pregnancy than those who are not in a healthy condition. It is true that drinking alcohol, smoking, and caffeine can negatively affect fertility. Being overweight or underweight can also affect fertility by interfering with hormone function.

- A national television commercial reminds us that *"an educated consumer is our best customer."* No where is the quote more meaningful than here. When you are knowledgeable about pregnancy and fertility you would know how to prepare your body and know what to ask your health care practitioner. Knowing and observing your fertility signs can tell you a lot about your body. Recording your basal body temperature and cervical fluid can help you pinpoint the best time to have intercourse while trying to conceive. These fertility signs can also reveal if you are ovulating regularly. Becoming familiar with your fertility will also help you discern between impending signs and symptoms of pregnancy.

- Visit your health care practitioner if you have not conceived after six months of purposeful intercourse. If you have not conceived after six months, contact your health care practitioner to discuss the possibility of fertility testing. Or you may decide to consult a fertility specialist at this time.

The Midlife Crisis

Over the years I have listened to hundreds of women as they shared with me their agonies on their midlife journey. They began to look back at their life expectations asking, "Is this all there is?" Her children are now in college or away from home and she is home all alone or with her husband, or her child has returned home after college. She has her family, the education, the car, the home, and the job but there is still something seemingly missing in her life. It is a thirst that material things cannot quench. They talk about an emptiness they feel inside that they are unable to shake. As I sit and listen, most will ask me, "Am I crazy?" The majority of these women are wonderful women in the best of shape but have this feeling of emptiness inside.

A lady named Rita said, *"I have given to my husband, my children, my job, my church, my community; when is somebody going to do something for me?"* Then came the tears. *"My husband doesn't care, my children don't listen to me, everyone takes, then asks for more. 'Give me . . . .' 'Give me . . . .' 'Do this for me.' They always want more of me. I don't know what else they want from me. I have nothing left to give. Maybe I am a fool?"*
"Why do you think you are a fool?" I asked.
"Because I allow everybody to use me."
"Rita, believe me, you are not a fool. I see you as a very strong, loving, and caring woman with the confidence to say, 'No' when needed. You are a woman who is trying to hold your family together. In doing so, you have surrendered your true self. You must remember, you don't have to give up who you truly are to gain his love."

Most women were trained to be givers. It is an unconscious behavior. Most women do not even know they have given up their soul, their desires, until what they have surrendered to no longer fit their needs. When she surrenders her authentic self to some temporary satisfaction that fulfills the expectations of others, e.g., mate, family, children, church or even society, to get the approval of others, she becomes become a "human doing" instead of a "human being." So she loses herself to get the approval of others. Getting the approval others results in a wonderful and euphoric feeling. She feels needed. She feels good; she feels loved. To meet their needs, however, she has become "Ms. Perfect" doing everything for everyone except herself.

This learned behavior starts very early in life and continues through adolescence and into adulthood. This behavior is fine if it is in tune with her temperament. She will not have any regrets. If it is not her temperament, this strategy can backfire and she will find herself right where she is now—feeling used. Also remember, at age thirty-five her estrogen level is not what it was when she was twenty-five. At twenty-five, her body was working with her and she thought of herself as superwoman. She had the energy then to take on the world, with no regard for who gave back to her. Now she is not quite as energetic as she was then. She has given to her family, community, church, and profession with little in return.

Another woman by the name of Eileen shared, *"I was scheduled for surgery. As I lay in my hospital bed being prepped for an operation, before being wheeled into the operating room, I actually freaked out as I began to reflect over my life. All of a sudden it hit me that anything could go wrong in the operating room, and what if I didn't make it? I have had other operations in the past and never had that reaction, I never freaked out before an operation. As they began to wheel me in, I was thinking, crying and praying 'O, My God'. I'm getting ready to go under the knife and I never really did anything for anyone but myself. I never got married or had children. I was told by others, even my own mother and father, that I was selfish and thought of no one but myself. I hurt the people who loved me. I am all by myself at thirty-seven. What will happen to my things? Who would be at my funeral? Not one person! My surgery was successful and I came out from under the knife, I asked God to change me. I realized that my life could have been over in a snap, I thank God for the revelation."*

I knew Eileen before her last operation and she was as she described-selfish and didn't care about anyone but herself. She emerged from her surgery a new and different person; very involved in her community and in the lives of others. She experienced an eye-opening midlife revelation. The midlife watershed years does not have to be negative. The reflection and subsequent questioning by some women causes a paradigm shift allowing her to see herself not as she is but as what she can become. So, if you are at that crossroad in your life and you have looked in the mirror and are not pleased with the image looking back at you because the image is not what you have dreamed of, it does not have to become your reality. It is time to change your position. I think it was Thomas Lifson, who said, "*Sometimes what you see really does depend on where you stand. Where you see yourself pinned in a box for years, you need to get out and stretch. Then say, 'I'm on my way out of here to someplace new. I'm taking the A train and I don't want anybody to follow me, let's go.'*" Maybe you cannot see the light at the end of the tunnel because of personal responsibilities, or you are stuck in a toxic marriage, but this is the time of life where some women are by themselves or with their children for several reasons. She might be separated, divorced, widowed or never married. Whatever it may be, you are not at the place you need to be.

Single Again

Dear Mr. Morgan,

After twenty-one years of marriage and four children I find myself divorced, alone and depressed. I am a professional woman with a very good salary, have a good job, and bad habits. Even though I know I am blessed to be where I am and have the things I have, I am still so alone. It seems that all I do is work, and come home to my kids, who are very seldom home. I find myself playing the X-Box for hours at a time, surfing the web, or maybe watching a movie on DVD or TV. I am happy I have my music. Without music, I would probably be in the mental institution. Music at home or in my car lifts my spirit.

I am becoming more and more depressed. I guess being single is part of the problem. All of my friends are married so we don't hangout like we used to. They don't call like they used too. The friends I would like to hang out with either moved or we lost touch. I have given my best to the only man I have ever really known. Before my divorce, I thought I would enjoy being at home alone, not answering to anyone. My thoughts have backfired on me. I find myself sinking deeper and deeper into emotional distress.

All this might be my fault. My father passed away two years ago, since then it has all been downhill. My ex kept asking me to speak to someone about my feelings. I went to one session of grief counseling. I left there feeling like crap, so I never went back. My ex and children continued the counseling; they seem to be fine. We were all close to my dad. My ex-husband never wanted the divorce, but again, I thought I would enjoy being at home alone, not answering to anyone, so he signed the papers.

Since my dad's death, I feel like I don't have anyone to talk to anymore, and that is killing me. A peace [sic] of me died with him. My only saving grace is that he said he was proud of me before he died, so I try to live my life to keep him proud of me. I withdrew from everyone after his death including my husband and my girls. I used to go to church but the people there were no help, other than wanting everything in my house after my divorce. There are several men who have asked me out but I wouldn't know what to do on a date. So why bother?

I still love my ex; I just feel that I was putting him through too much after my father's death. I love my home, but it is empty. I wish I had never gone through the divorce. I think I should probably seek your help. Maybe you can help me with my depression. Or maybe introduce me to someone to just have fun, start a relationship and eventually fall in love. But, then again, I guess that is what we are all looking for. It is too bad I don't have the balls to actually get out there and do it.

Please help me,
Ms. Brown

At our first meeting we discussed Ms. Brown's letter and decided upon a six-session course of therapeutic action that involved her girls, and if we could, her ex-husband. She enthusiastically agreed. At the end of the sixth session, Ms. Brown not only had her family back but also had her life back. Her husband loved and wanted to be in his wife's life, but wanted to give her space in the hope that she would come to the realization her problem was not with him or their marriage but with her emotional attachment with her deceased dad. Our counseling concentration is now about the loss of her father. Ms. Brown is again enjoying life.

The Loss of Your Authentic Self

"I am thirty-nine and after being married for twenty years, my husband left me for someone else. I have so many mixed emotions that always seem to include anger, loneliness, isolation, embarrassment, frustration and failure, but most of all anger. I gave him the best that I had, including two children, Brenda and Olivia. I am still wondering what happened? Why did he leave? Our home was a loving one; we all did things together. I find myself all alone; our daughters are away at college. Everyone is wondering why, how and what will I do now that my divorced is final. No one could possibly understand how I feel. I don't know if I am going to survive this. Everybody is telling me it takes time and I am going to be fine. I am not going to be fine, I can't start over. I feel betrayed, lonely, confused and angry. Don't tell me how many women feel alone, betrayed and angry after their divorce. I was a very good wife and mother. I didn't deserve this."
BJ, Brooklyn

When I read her story, like so many others sharing her hopelessness with no light at the end of the tunnel, I see a woman who has given up her authentic self.

"If you haven't found it yet, keep looking. Don't settle. As with all matters of the heart, you'll know when you find it. And, like any great relationship, it just gets better and better as the years roll on."—Steve Jobs

Too many women lose touch with themselves early on. As little girls, they tried eagerly to please the people around them. To be honest, sometimes it was much easier to go along with whatever their parents wanted. If her expressed opinions or desires differed from theirs, a conflict ensued, so it was easier to go along with them by keeping quiet. Mom and Dad made all the decisions—what to wear to school, what to eat for dinner, what movie to see. She becomes lost, not knowing what she wants in life.

Many women, like BJ, who got married at twenty and passed the decision-making on to their husband. It wasn't until after her divorce (after twenty years of marriage) that she realized how much she had lost touch with herself. She has a hard time making the simplest decisions: how she wants to spend her time, where to go for dinner, where to live, what kind of car to buy, where to travel. She wasn't used to having choices or thinking about what she really wanted.

She had no idea who she was now that she was no longer a wife and mother and daughter. During her marriage, she paid many of the costs of being unauthentic: she was unassertive, she avoided conflict, she was always trying to please others. As wife and mother, she had learned to subjugate her own needs to the demands of her children and her busy husband. When she became single, she found it hard to know what her needs were. It has taken her years of self-observation and self-assessment, therapy, coaching, and training to find out what she really needs and wants. She often found herself paralyzed with making a decision or she felt anxious when she was in a conflict with a friend. After months of working with her, she still wanted to please others. The difference is that now she notices when she was doing it and that motivates her to be more authentic.

Age may also play a factor in BJ becoming authentic. As she got older she was less worried about what other people thought; she didn't need to please others as she did before. I was able to make her realize that the time to be real is now or never. If she wanted to be authentic, now was the time. It was time to realize that one and only unique person she was. Being authentic takes more than being aware; authenticity demands action. *Being authentic means being congruent with one's inner awareness and outer behavior.* It takes courage to be authentic. To be authentic often means expressing unpopular opinions and taking unpopular actions; to be authentic can create disharmony and conflict because of the risk of disapproval or loss of relationships. Yet not living an authentic life means losing yourself, creating inner disharmony and inner conflict. Ultimately this disharmony is harder to live with. I have become convinced of this.

Being in relationship with significant others, friends and family can bring out our authenticity, or not. I believe that we all have within us buds of our authentic potential. Each relationship we are in will connect with our dormant buds and can cause them to grow and blossom. A woman's relationships can help her grow into her authenticity or they can squelch her growth. She needs to become more aware of the influence of her relationships. She should try to speak up more often when her needs are in conflict; she must try to voice her needs and wants immediately when she is aware of them. She will notice that she has attracted more friends who are authentic themselves. Their courage to be authentic will inspire her and they will also encourage and support her in her efforts to be authentic.

Having authentic role models can help her know how to be authentic. You can find role models in church, books, politicians, communities, and in leadership roles. You can find them if you look around. Unfortunately, women suffer from having few authentic role models, in life or in books. In history books, there is a notable absence of women heroines. In novels, there is an invisibility of the female character, which creates a sense of powerlessness and actively undermines self-confidence. Women role models are out there, but they must be sought. *When the student is ready, the teacher will appear.*

Cultivating Your Authentic Self

Start with describing your Self:

- Who am I, really?
- What are your physical attributes and abilities?
- What are your roles? Who are you in each of your roles? (e.g., mother, daughter, sister, teacher, etc.)

- What are your characteristics?
- What are your skills?
- What are your competencies? (characteristics + skills = what is special and unique about you)
- What are your talents?
- What are your preferences?
- What is important to you?
- What are your values?
- What are your needs?
- What are your wants?
- What are your interests?
- What are your goals and dreams?
- What brings you passion?
- What is your life purpose?

It would help if you asked your significant other, colleagues or family members to answer the above questions, too. *How would they describe you?*

Now, you may or may not be ready to leave your marriage. Sometimes what happens is that there is an intense soul hunger going on on the inside. I've had to explain this to so many women who give themselves away to get the love of their mate. Too many have failed to develop their own identity in the process of learning how to do for and take care of others. Many women give up or give away various parts of themselves to keep a relationship. It is also true that what attracted them to their mate was perhaps what they had not yet opened to or accepted in themselves. Although the process may be difficult, owning their authentic self is one of the gifts that can emerge from the pain of divorce. It takes courage for them to reclaim those elements of themselves that they were willing to sacrifice to make their marriage work. For example, while they were married, they may have given up being proficient around the house by acting as though they were incapable; or they may have denied their intellectual capacity by not finishing college. Some wives do this primarily because they are afraid of out pacing their husbands. In an effort to please their mate, they may have given up all their "free time" instead of pursuing activities they enjoyed.

Perhaps they felt the relationship should have been completely symbiotic, so they abandoned personal friends of long-standing, or failed to develop friendships of their own outside the marriage. Whatever it was, it was a denial of their authentic self.

I am not talking here about compromise, we all compromise. Compromise is an important and necessary part of living with another person. I am talking about the tendency to completely deny or let go of important aspects of her essential self. The predicament some women find themselves in during the watershed stage is that of reclaiming herself and struggling to keep it alive, to become what she was before she gave in (or gave way) to the (entanglement) relationship.

Reclaiming Your Identity And Authentic Self

Sometimes I ask women during the watershed stage who they are, and most respond by giving me their name. A name does not say very much about who a person is, it is similar to an address. It identifies you from another person but it says very little about who you are. Most of these women identify with their roles and not themselves even when these roles may have changed. They may say, "I am a wife, homemaker or a mother." It would be good for her to ask herself, "Who am I now, if I'm not a wife?" "What parts of my identity did I bury in my mate?" When you disown or dishonor your true Self and do not take the time to reclaim your Self, you give up your self-worth. You limit the possibility of intimacy in future relationships. Many of you never recognized or celebrated yourselves as being truly unique and distinct to begin with. You surrendered to everyone but yourself (your mate, your children, your parents, your job, your degree, etc.), so now allow yourself to be a part of another person without giving yourself away. Give yourself the opportunity to know the authentic you. You are a unique, one of a kind, never to be repeated child of God.

When you give up so much of your authentic Self, there is a subtle erosion of self-worth and of the soul, and gradually who you really are completely disappears. The person your mate initially was attracted to does not exist anymore. You abandon yourself—and your mate abandons you.

As you become capable of being honest about who you are, rather than hiding and trying to please others, you become increasingly able to accept the truth about others. That does not mean you choose someone with whom you are not compatible. It means that when you openly make yourself present and available, you can receive and be received by someone with whom your heart will sing.

During my divorce recovery workshops, I invite participants to list five things they gave up in order to be in a relationship with their mate. Often at the top of their list would be people, friends, hobbies, pursuits, feelings, possessions, religion, etc. Invariably, one of the most repeated items on the list are—friends. Other frequently listed items are-personal and/or spiritual growth and time alone for myself. It's sad, but true, that many of the women I've encountered in this process are aware that, for some reason, their relationships have produced a prolonged period of stagnation in the area of personal/ spiritual growth—a period of non-growth and non-creativity that is most important to recover and nurture. The second part of the exercise is to go back and write under each item what you are doing now (or would like to do) to reclaim those things. If the woman married very young, then she may have failed to have developed her own identity in the process of learning how to do for and take care of others.

Now midlife is as good a time as any other to begin to reevaluate your own life. When your estrogen level begins to fade, you begin to look at things and do things differently. Your blinders are off and for most of you there is light at the end of the tunnel. So now that you can see a bit clearer do not neglect the other people in your life. Make your life a priority, but the people and things that God has blessed to be with you on your journey should have a place in your life, too. Let them know your needs and how you need to be loved. Paint a picture filled with details so that the other person doesn't have to fill in the blanks.

Now think for a moment. Do you know what love is? Do you know how you want someone to love you? Let me give you some insight. As soon as you realize that your Love Bank balance needs to be refilled, you should ask yourself, *"What could this man do for me that would make me the happiest woman in this world?"* That very question focuses on a core issue in marriage—the issue of care. I could have asked the question, "How would you like this man to care for you?" As it turns out, "care" in marriage is doing what it takes to make each other happy.

When you were married, you and your husband both promised to care for each other, and you expected that care from each other. You were infatuated and you were highly motivated to make each other happy, or as happy as infatuation could make you. It might not have occurred to you at the time that if you didn't care for each other the right way, it might never grow into the love you both expected and needed. And along with your loss of love, you might lose your willingness to care for each other.

At the time, infatuation had no idea what caring for each other the right way was. To care the right way, you both must make Love Bank deposits. I have found that the best way to make those deposits is to meet each other's most important emotional needs. What is an emotional need? It is a craving that, when satisfied, leaves you with a feeling of happiness and contentment; and when unsatisfied, leaves you with a feeling of unhappiness and frustration. There are probably thousands of emotional needs. A need for a new house, a new car, a vacation, I could go on and on. Some people have some of those needs while others have different needs. If you feel good about doing something, or if someone does something for you that makes you feel good, an emotional need has been met. But not all emotional needs are created equally. When some emotional needs are met, you may feel comfortable. But when all of your emotional needs are met, your Love Bank becomes full and a full Love Bank will make you feel downright euphoric. In fact, it will make you so happy that you're likely to fall in love with the person that filled your Love Bank. I call these our most important emotional needs because they make the largest Love Bank deposits of all, and those are the very same emotional needs that a husband and wife expect each other to meet in marriage. You may need to proceed cautiously if your husband is insecure, but always remember, these are your needs and you should not be afraid to have them met.

Financial Strategies During Your Transitional Or Watershed Journey

The majority of women in my counsel is in a financial swamp, barely keeping their head above water, living from paycheck to paycheck, borrowing from relatives and friends in between and has credit card debt that is out of control. During the watershed years, most women are in their transitional years financially also. If you're in this category or facing new life challenges, perhaps recently widowed, divorced, married, (or about to be) diagnosed or dealing with an illness; then you're a woman in transition, and you have special financial needs.

You may be receiving conflicting advice from family and friends. You may be struggling with grief, guilt or other powerful emotions. You may even feel strapped for time or feel as if each day is an eternity, but life goes on. At this time, your personal finances may not be a priority although it should be. If your finances are in disarray, you are "handcuffed" and will not be able to move forward in your transitional journey. It may be difficult to finish your transition.

Although each woman's particular circumstances are different, women in transition always face certain issues in common. Let's begin with financial strategies for the similarities and then address specific transitional situations.

Numbness, Denial, Impulsiveness And Conflicting Advice

Women in transition often report feeling as if they're moving through a thick fog, or as if their brain is numb or filled with cotton candy. You are not alone in feeling this way. It's a basic human coping or self-protection mechanism to shield ourselves from an onslaught of stressful events and emotions. The danger is when this numbness extends to shielding us from responding to the consequences of our financial behaviors. The denial reflected in months of unpaid bills and overdue notices can quickly destroy a lifetime of credit-worthiness and take years to recover from. Impulsive decisions like purchasing expensive vacations or gifts, or hastily buying or selling major assets like your business, home, or stock portfolio can leave you with major regrets, tax liabilities, and a diminished net worth for years to come. Meanwhile, it can seem as if you're in a vortex of swirling, conflicting advice from friends and families about what you should or shouldn't do about your situation.

Given these widespread reactions and experiences, certain financial strategies work for nearly every woman in transition:

- **Buy time.** If you did not previously prepare for this stage of life, you may want to defer all essential decisions to a professional. You may want to seek professional financial advice on what decisions simply cannot be deferred, but in general you want to buy time in order to work your way through this life transition. If keeping on top of your monthly paperwork and chores is an issue, you may want to consider the services of a personal concierge or bookkeeper.
- **Buy flexibility.** Now is not the time to commit all your cash to long-term investments or pay off your mortgage. Think of any slightly diminished returns during this period as the price of flexibility. A year in the future, your needs may be quite different so your goal now is to preserve options for your soon-to-be changed lifestyle. Again, objective professional financial advice may be helpful.
- **Take care of yourself.** Thoughtful financial decisions are more likely when you are well rested and at peace with your life stage. Eating healthy, making time in your calendar for a daily walk or other physical exercise, and carving out time for quiet rituals of meditation, warm baths and other soothing activities are proven coping techniques for the stresses of major life transitions. Studies demonstrate that taking care

of yourself in such ways can provide wellness and other important benefits with little cost or risk.

Acknowledge your vulnerability. Many women broadcast their emotional vulnerability during a life transition without being aware of it. Unfortunately, there are unscrupulous people who will take advantage of your vulnerability. Once you acknowledge your vulnerability and are willing to protect yourself from unscrupulous people you will be ahead of the game. It is especially important to be careful about the people and services you engage to help you. Please utilize any and all community resources for women in transition.

In addition to the challenges shared in common by nearly every woman in transition, specific transitional situations can also bring financial challenges and traps.

Divorce

Whether you are considering separation or are already in the divorce process, you will be making decisions that will affect the rest of your life. Dividing up assets in a divorce has never been an easy task, but increasingly complex investment options make it even harder now. Dividing a stock portfolio the wrong way can trigger vastly unequal tax consequences. Overlooking the QDRO form (pronounced *"KWA-dro"*) can make a mess of dividing retirement plan assets. You may need help navigating the economic aspects of a divorce, as opposed to the legal issues such as custody that are handled by divorce lawyers. Divorce can stimulate a sense of loss and grief. Here are some strategies to safeguard your finances during and after a divorce:

Keep taxes in mind. A stock portfolio split down the middle might not be financially equal.

Don't be house poor. Many divorcing women want to keep their homes for emotional reasons and to provide stability for their kids, but maintaining a house also means mortgage, tax and upkeep expenses.

Know the financial consequences of splitting up retirement plans. They involve tricky tax rules, so be sure you have the proper paperwork and talk to qualified advisors.

Update your wills, trusts, and beneficiary designations on retirement plans and insurance policies so your ex or some other unintended beneficiary doesn't end up inheriting a windfall.

How To Avoid Financial Traps During Illness

- Whether you or a family member has recently been diagnosed with a serious illness, you will be facing many new challenges and decisions. Serious illness can stimulate grieving for the loss of the healthy, able-bodied self you've always known.
- Establish a power of attorney. A power of attorney needs to be drafted so someone can handle your financial affairs while you are incapacitated.
- Choose your health care proxy. If you have just received a diagnosis for a life-threatening condition or terminal illness, you want someone you trust empowered to authorize or decline medical procedures.
- Consider establishing a trust so the assets you managed during your lifetime pass to your heirs as you intended, without the stress, expense and time delay of the probate process.

How To Avoid Financial Traps Before You Say "I Do" Again

- Second marriages and blended families bring the financial challenge of caring for each other and for multiple beneficiaries.
- Update wills, trusts and beneficiary designations on retirement plans and insurance, so both of you, your children and his children are cared for as you both intend.

- Discuss your finances. Know how much debt your partner has and the impact of your option to share or combine finances. Do this before you say "I do."

How To Avoid Financial Traps During Grief or Loss

- Although grief resulting from the death of someone you love is readily acknowledged, many women are surprised to experience grief from the loss of their health, or the loss of a love, or divorce. Avoid grief-driven decision-making. Sometimes guilt intrudes itself in our lives when we inherit gifts or insurance claim money from our lost loved one who has transitioned. This guilt can lead to foolish spending, or simply giving away what was intended to provide for your financial security. To avoid this, be thankful for the time you and your loved one had to spend together and how they thought enough of your relationship to leave you their love in the form of a gift.
- Avoid making decisions by default. Not looking at your finances can cause unintended outcomes and missed opportunities, or unintended tax issues.

Nutritional Needs For The Watershed Years

Midlife is when many women begin to experience breakdowns of their bodies. It need not be that way if she follows a healthy lifestyle to protect her body's healing system and maintain optimal health as she ages. Aging is a natural process and it is a normal part of maturing.

The most effective approach to long life is the foundation of a women's health: a deliberate diet, enjoyable exercise, rest and relaxation, herbs and nutrients targeted to hormonal balance, and solid emotional support. I've seen these combinations make all the difference with our female clients. In our earlier example, Ms. Carter received some comprehensive testing looking at all aspects of the hormonal axis including hypothalamus, pituitary, thyroid, adrenal, and ovarian function. Women who experience hormone imbalance range in age from nineteen to sixty years of age. I would recommend a full medical examination by a competent physician be done before commencing any of these therapies.

Exercise can help you take charge of your health and maintain the level of fitness necessary for an active, independent lifestyle. Many women think that physical decline is an inevitable consequence of aging. For the most part, this is not true. Much of the physical frailty attributed to aging is actually the result of inactivity, disease, or poor nutrition. The good news is that many problems can be helped or even reversed by improving lifestyle behaviors. One of the major benefits of regular physical activity is protection against coronary heart disease, the number one killer of many women.

Physical activity also provides some protection against other chronic diseases such as adult-onset diabetes, arthritis, hypertension, certain cancers, osteoporosis, and depression. In addition, research has proven that exercise can ease tension and reduce the amount of stress one feels. Simply put, exercise is one of the best things you can do for your health. At the same time you should start with a pharmaceutical-grade multivitamin-mineral complex, like my *Perfect Food Plus Formula*, to provide the key levels of micronutrients your body requires, which are often lacking in the American diets. This formula targeted nutritional support may be enough to begin healing your hormonal pathways.

I would also suggest our *Female Balance* and *Female Formula* as your second step. These herbal equilibrium formulas are especially formulated for women transitioning through perimenopause. Medicinal herbs support the body's ability to restore hormonal balance by mimicking hormonal actions at a molecular level. They also interact with the body's tissues to facilitate natural hormone regulation. Most women find that adding high-quality nutrients and phytotherapy is enough. Others need more support to reach ideal symptom relief. This can mean adding more essential fatty acids, or amino acids like 5-HTP, or complementary therapies like acupuncture or chiropractic, just to name a few possibilities. Different women have different needs, so she may want to work with a health care practitioner to decide which added therapies would be the best for her.

Your Spiritual Journey is Different, But It Continues

As a woman's spiritual journey continues, she will change in many ways. She may notice that her traditional paradigm no longer provides the spiritual haven it once did. She may also notice that the places and people she once felt close to no longer bring the warmth and security she now needs. This journey may take her into personal areas of her own life she neglected in years past.

She is not the same woman she was ten years ago or even two years ago! Her needs have changed. God should not be the same to her now as He was to her last year. Her needs from Him are different just as her needs from Him were different from when she was a little girl. She has faced many challenges and has had to twist and turn to accommodate and survive as He helped her to navigate through the maze of her life. As she gets older, God will reveal His secret universal laws to her in order to make her ongoing journey easier. Remember the power of the Divine is the only power where the victim mentality is removed from her life and she is standing in her own God-given power. This power helps her to decide deliberately what course she desires her life to take. Her spiritual journey is never ending as she is constantly evolving. If she is to progress as a human being, then she must advance her own spiritual practices.

Her biggest challenge, in my opinion, is to remember that she is a spiritual being having a human experience, instead of a human being having a spiritual experience. It has taken me many years to understand fully what I have gone through over the years. Many doors to the spiritual world have been opened to me and now I can share this experience with you. The experience of knowing one's true authentic self, or the remembering of who one truly is, signifies the beginning of one's spiritual journey. By focusing on her spiritual life, a woman's daily interaction with others will be welcoming and relaxing and her life will be at peace. To have this peace within, she must first forgive and ask for forgiveness to those she has wronged or those who have wronged her. If she accepts the One and only God of her creation and then accepts herself and her life, and practices this way of life, it will soon become a part of who she really is: one with God and the universe.

Questioning Choices In Life

Questioning choices in life is inevitable. Dwelling in regret, indecision, and doubt does not work. Being defined as someone who lives in the past isn't fun. If you continually look back and say, "I should have or if only I had . . ." you are not progressing or showing gratitude. I have a friend who was always looking back; she was angry, blaming others, sickly, and looking for handouts. One day I got tired of the conversations about her decisions and what life would have looked like had she made different choices. I said to her, "You cannot dwell there, if you do life will be to you a terrible master. Those things are in the past, it's time to move on." After spending time in counsel with her, she is beginning to change her paradigm now. I can see her progressively gaining love and favor from others and accepting herself. She is also thankful for her life.

There has been some research conducted by Dr. Rick Nauert that determined that over analyzing and second-guessing one's decisions can lead to stress and unhappiness. Psychologists have termed individuals who obsess over decisions—big or small—and then fret about their choices later as "maximizers." "Satisfiers," on the other hand, tend to make a decision and then live with it.

A new study sheds light on why it is difficult for some to make a decision that they can be happy with. Dr. Joyce Ehrlinger, an assistant professor of psychology at Florida State University, said that individuals usually fall between the extremes. In fact, there's a whole continuum of ways people avoid commitment without really avoiding it. Ehrlinger's research on decision-making is found in the journal

Personality and Individual Differences. The paper examines whether "maximizers show less commitment to their choices than satisfiers in a way that leaves them less satisfied with their choices." Ehrlinger and her research team discovered maximizers' tendency to focus on finding the best option ultimately undermines their commitment to their final choices. (Source: Florida State University December 16, 2011)

Amanda has two older and one younger sister who were raised by their mother, Mrs. Hilliard. Their mother struggled with drugs and prostitution all of their lives. Amanda was raised by her Aunt Zola, who gave her the best of everything-home, clothing, education, and culture. Amanda grew up to be an attorney with a successful law firm in New York City; while both her older sisters became drug addicts and her younger sister was arrested for prostitution on several occasions. Amanda visited my office, complaining that her mother gave her away, did not like her, and only cared for her sisters. She resented her mother for giving her to her aunt. She also resented her Aunt Zola for not allowing her mother to raise her. Amanda felt she would have been better off raised by her mother until I turned on the light by asking her three questions.

> *"Who raised your sisters?" I asked.*
> *"My mother," she said.*
> *"How are they doing?" I countered.*
> *"They are drug addicts and prostitutes, like my mother," she responded.*
> *"With that in mind, what would have happened to you if your mother had raised you?" I continued.*
> *"Wow! Most likely I would be like my sisters," she concluded.*

I instructed Amanda to please call her mother and thank her for allowing her aunt to raise her. I told her to call her aunt next and to thank her for the love, care, and support she gave to her over the years. I advised her to stop looking back and to decide from today forward to look ahead, not behind her.

Always remember that choices in life are made with good intentions at the time of decision. If you could go back and change them, you might decide in a very different way. However, we cannot go backward; only forward. There are people who engaged in addictive habits who continually look back at the problems they caused in their lives. If you are one of these people, make it as right as possible, forgive yourself, forgive others, and move on. Look forward to the exciting journey ahead. There are adventures that you have not experienced. There are happy moments and joy-jumping hours that you will possibly miss if you keep looking back. Do not miss them; you will certainly regret losing those beautiful moments ahead. We are all entitled to reminisce. We are all entitled to wonder fleetingly if our lives would have been happier, healthier or more adventuresome if we had chosen a different lifestyle. We might have traveled more, visited the world, or became more educated if we had chosen different paths. Would your mate have been the same? Would your life have been better? Would you have moved to other regions of the country, or would other and better opportunities have come your way?

You Shape Your Life By The Choices You Make

Most women forget the great power they hold within to shape their lives. Your life is shaped by the choices you make. You are the only one who can choose how to live your life or create your life's path. Your first step is to choose the type of life path you want, whether valleys, hills, or rolling plains. Know that you ultimately make the choice.

Ask yourself: *What does it look like? How does it feel? How do I create a life path?* Start by visualizing the life you really would like. Write down and describe in detail your vision so it becomes alive and real for you. You may spend a great deal of time creating the perfect path for yourself; but there are two things you should remember: 1) Life is never perfect. 2) The road you take might become bumpy, painful, or joyful because of the choices you make along the way.

There may be times that the choices you make cause your path to become bumpy, confusing and/or uncertain. It may seem like a series of hills and valleys; you may never experience any balance. When this happens, you should stop and examine the choices you made that have taken you down this path. You should evaluate those choices and identify alternative (or new) choices that will bring you back to the path you originally envisioned. Remember again, we shape our lives by the choices we make.

Despite the wise choices you made in creating your path, you cannot control the unexpected. Some things may hit you from the blind side. Although you may not expect the unexpected, you should plan for it. You can either choose to give up, or keep going and turn the situation from negative to positive. Spend your energy looking for positive solutions and don't waste your time focusing on the problem. That is negative energy that will get you nowhere fast. Once again, the choices you make help to shape your life. Each choice will have a different effect on your life. The choice is yours. Positive energy focused on solutions tends to bring positive results in all aspects of life. The results can take the form of happiness, satisfaction, inner peace, humility, gratitude or just a sense of accomplishment that somehow increases your self-esteem and gives you greater self-confidence. When you choose to turn the bumps in the road into successful experiences, you reach new levels of success and enhance your overall quality of life. In fact it is these choices that may inspire you and positively transform your life.

The secret to making wise choices is based on your values, morals, principles, and self-awareness. Choices should not be based purely on your emotions. The wiser approach is to consider the state of your emotions when you make choices. The best choices are made when you recognize and understand your emotions and use this awareness to manage yourself, your choices, and relationships with others. The ability to understand your emotions and the emotions of others is an important skill to have when making choices.

Be yourself. Trying to be anyone else is a waste of the person you are. Embrace that individual inside you that has ideas, strengths, and beauty like no one else. Be the person you know yourself to be—the best version of you—on your terms. Above all, be true to you: if you cannot put your heart in it, take yourself out of it.

Carol Giannantonio is a certified life coach, who has helped thousands of people reach their full potential and create the life they love. She has given us 14 points to help us find our lives.

1. **Get your priorities straight.** Twenty years from now it won't really matter what shoes you wore today, how your hair looked, or what brand of jeans you bought. What will matter is how you loved, what you learned, and how you applied this knowledge.

2. **Take full responsibility for your goals.** If you really want good things in your life to happen, you have to make them happen yourself. You can't sit around and hope that somebody else will help you. You have to make your own future and not think that your destiny is tied to the actions and choices of others.

3. **Know your worth.** When someone treats you like you're just one of many options, help them narrow their choice by removing yourself from the equation. Sometimes you have to try not to care, no matter how much you do. Sometimes you can mean almost nothing to someone who means so much to you. It's not pride; it's self-respect. Don't expect to see positive changes in your life if you surround yourself with negative people. Don't give part-time people a full-time position in your life. Know your value and what you have to offer, and never settle for anything less than what you deserve.

4. **Choose the right perspective.** Perspective is everything. When faced with long check-out lines, traffic jams, or waiting an hour past your appointment time, you have two choices: You can get frustrated and enraged, or you can view it as life's way of giving you a guilt-free breather from rushing, and spend that time daydreaming, conversing, or watching the

clouds. The first choice will raise your blood pressure. The second choice will raise your consciousness.

5. **Don't let your old problems punish your dreams.** Learn to let go of things you can't control. The next time you're tempted to rant about a situation that you think ended unfairly, remind yourself of this: You'll never kill off your anger by beating the story to death. So close your mouth, unclench your fists, and redirect your thoughts. When left untended, the anger will slowly wither, and you'll be left to live in peace as you grow toward a better future.

6. **Choose the things that truly matter.** Some things just don't matter much—like the kind of car you drive. How big of a deal is that in the grand scheme of life? Not a big deal at all. But lifting a person's heart? Now, that matters. The whole problem with most people is, they KNOW what matters, but they don't CHOOSE it. They get distracted. They don't put first things first. The hardest and smartest way to live is choosing what truly matters, and pursuing it passionately. *Suggested Reading: The 7 Habits of Highly Effective People by Steven Covey*

7. **Love YOU.** Let someone love you just the way you are—as flawed as you might be, as unattractive as you sometimes feel, and as unaccomplished as you think you are. Yes, let someone love you despite all of this; and let that someone be YOU. *Suggested Reading: Food for Thought 25 Ways to Protect Yourself from Disease and Promote Excellent Health by Dr. Ray Morgan*

8. **Accept your strengths and weaknesses.** Be confident being YOU. We often waste too much time comparing ourselves to others, and wishing to be something we're not. Everybody has their own strengths and weaknesses, and it is only when we accept everything we are, and aren't, that we are able to become who we are capable of being.

9. **Stand up for YOU.** You were born to be real, not to be perfect. You're here to be YOU, not to be what someone else wants you to be. Stand up for yourself, look them in the eye, and say, "Don't judge me until you know me, don't underestimate me until you challenge me, and don't talk about me until you've talked to me."

10. **Learn from others, and move on when you must.** You can't expect to change people. Either you accept who they are, or you start living your life without them. And just because something ends, doesn't mean it never should have been. You lived, you learned, you grew, and you moved on. Some people come into your life as blessings; others come into your life as lessons.

11. **Be honest in your relationships.** Don't cheat! If you're not happy, be honest, and move on if you must. When you're truly in love, being faithful isn't a sacrifice; it's a joy.

12. **Get comfortable with being uncomfortable.** Life as we know it can change in a blink of an eye. Unlikely friendships can blossom, important careers can be tossed aside and a long lost hope can be rekindled. It might feel a little uncomfortable at times, but know that life begins at the end of your comfort zone. So if you're feeling uncomfortable right now, know that the change taking place in your life is not an ending, but a new beginning. *Suggested Reading: The Power of Full Engagement by Jim Loehr and Tony Schwartz*

13. **Be who you were born to be.** Don't get to the end of your life and find that you lived only the length of it; live the width of it as well. When it comes to living as a passionate, inspired human being, the only challenge greater than learning to walk a mile in someone else's shoes, is learning to walk a lifetime comfortably in your own. Follow your heart, and take your brain with you. When you are truly comfortable in your own skin, not everyone will like you, but you won't care about it one bit.

14. **Never give up on YOU.** This is your life; shape it, or someone else will. Strength shows not only in the ability to hold on, but in the ability to start over when you must. It is never too late to become what you might have been. *"Keep learning, adapting, and growing. You may not be there yet, but you are closer than you were yesterday."*

Remember, you will only be remembered for two things: The problems you caused and the problems you solved for others.

Sex In Your Watershed Years

I have counseled some women in their forties who believed their bodies and sex are taboo, unclean, and a certain pathway to everlasting hell. They may not have had the best sex education when they were younger, but certainly with the advent of the internet and the loosening of standards and ethics on American television, they must have learned something about their bodies and sex in the last twenty or so years. Girls mature much faster than boys do, and unlike men, they savor the journey and hit their strides in their forties. Funny, how this coincides with the new term, "cougar." Men spend from the ages of sixteen to twenty-five with their pelvises in constant motion, emulating a jack hammer whenever the opportunity presents itself. Women, on the other hand can endure for years. You don't need the stimulants to get you going.

In life's great ironic twists, men do learn this and slow down just in time for your libidos to go haywire and long for the jack hammer days. Is it any wonder the rate of incompatibility when a couple reaches their forties? Men want to go slow and younger girls are eager for the opportunity to take an older lover. Why not, all the men her age are still boys, hammering away at it. Meanwhile, what about the woman in her forties? Well, "jack hammers" are starting to look good again and with good reason. He can keep up with her lust for fulfillment, does not need pharmaceuticals to rise to the occasion, and unless he neglected his body, most forty-year-old men work out and try to take care of themselves and look good all together. Now back to the original line of thinking.

Now it is socially acceptable for a woman to be as open and real about her sexuality more than ever before. Just a mere ten years ago, it was still a man's world when it came to sex. It was perfectly normal for a man to hit midlife crisis, get a divorce, a fast car, and a twenty year-old to go with it, but it was not so for women. So ladies, if you are lacking in sexual knowledge, please, book a party, buy a book on Amazon and have it delivered in a plain brown wrapper, (that will be our secret), or ask a friend. I don't think you will burn in hell for that. So, be happy, be excited and be curious.

Chapter Seven

STAGE FOUR-THE CLIMACTERIC SEASON OF CHANGE (AGES 45-55)

A Time When The Reproductive System Physically Shuts Down

Congratulations women, for arriving at a wonderful stage of life. Most women may not think so, but the journey has been long. Although the journey continues, you are at a good place—menopause or postmenopause. Again congratulations!

Menopause is the term used for the last menstrual period a woman will ever have, and is commonly known as the "change of life". The truth is there are many similarities between having a period and menopause. The menopause phase of a woman's life typically occurs at the average age of 51, give or take a few years. There are two kinds of menopause and premature menopause. *Perimenopause* is the period of years in a woman's life leading up to menopause when the body produces lesser amounts of hormones sometimes resulting in physical and emotional symptoms. Premature menopause usually happens prior to the age of 40 for reasons such as surgical removal of the ovaries or damaged ovaries as a result of cancer treatments, causing an immediate onset.

If you were to compare a menstrual period, PMS, and menopause in a woman's life, you would see that many of the symptoms are the same. The symptoms include a combination of psychological, emotional, and physical changes, including mood swings, mood depression, oversensitivity, memory problems, migraine headaches, memory loss, muscle aches, hot flashes, heart palpitations, lack of concentration. Again, estrogen and progesterone control a woman's menopause and period, preparing the body for pregnancy every month. When pregnancy does not occur, her body releases an egg and she has a period. This reduced level of those hormones is what produces the symptoms of menopause. Again, menopause is simply a stage of life when the hormone levels in a woman's body lower. These are some of the factors menopause and a woman's period have in common.

Lifestyle Changes

A woman's lifestyle changes and other treatments can have an impact during both phases of menopause. For instance, she should include regular exercise, eat healthy foods, avoid excessive salt, sugar, caffeine, and alcohol and make sure the body gets enough vitamins, amino acids, omega-3s, and minerals to remain healthy. A clear understanding of menopause and a period is so important for both stages of menopause. As said before, there are many changes that occur in a woman's body. Because of this, it is a time of life that can be confusing or seem mysterious for some women, yet these changes in life can bring a sense of freedom by just being knowledgeable.

The Climacteric Period

This climacteric period, the time of menopause, is called "*the change.*" Now understand what menopause is. Menopause is nothing but the cessation of the menses. I remember asking one of my clients if she knew how long a woman is in menopause. She replied, "Until God brings you out." When I told her that menopause was only for a day. She quickly stated, "No, I have had menopause for five years."

As previously stated, menopause is the actual cessation or the stopping of the menstrual cycle. This occurs on a single day. After that one day, you are in *postmenopause*. Any time before that is *premenopause*. Why then do we use_the words menopause and postmenopause interchangeably?

The premenopausal period can last ten years, usually from age forty to fifty. That is the average length of time. Somewhere between those ages is usually when the first signs of a decrease in the estrogen level occurs. That first sign could be an irregular period, or it could be just one single hot flash. You may not feel another one for another five years. At the time you have the one hot flash, it starts your premenopausal period. After that you will begin to get a fluctuation in your estrogen level. Like the watershed years, when your estrogen level drops, it will do so gradually. It does not mean that you can't become pregnant. It just means that you will get a fluctuation in your estrogen level to the extent that you begin to feel some or all of the following symptoms.

Postmenopausal Symptoms

Usually the symptoms associated with menopause die down in some women once she reaches the postmenopausal stage. There have been cases when some women continue to experience certain symptoms even during the postmenopausal stage. The main reason for this is because of the hormonal changes that occur during her menopausal stage. During this time, estrogen and progesterone levels go down, giving rise to several symptoms. Sometimes, the symptoms may occur due to some underlying health problem and hence, it is important to see a health practitioner for a complete and detailed examination before doing anything else.

Vaginal Bleeding

One of the symptoms seen often in postmenopausal women is vaginal bleeding. Most of the time this bleeding is harmless; and is due to hormonal imbalance. However, it can also be a sign of something serious in the reproductive system. Hence, if you experience vaginal bleeding after not having periods for twelve months continuously, consult your health practitioner immediately.

Vaginal Dryness and Itching

Feeling the need to scratch the vagina frequently is another symptom that is attached to the postmenopause stage. Constant itching in the vaginal area can lead to a burning sensation in that area. Vaginal dryness can also be experienced along with the sensation of itching. Dryness in the vaginal area can become the reason for lack of sexual interest in many women. Your health practitioner can recommend a lubricant to get rid of the problem of vaginal dryness as well as itching. However, these may have some long term side effects and hence, it is advisable to use home remedies like olive oil for curing this problem.

Hot Flashes

Another common postmenopausal symptom is hot flashes, which can be accompanied with heart palpitations and night sweats. If you are postmenopausal, you may have hot flashes not only at night but also in the day, and it may last for not more than a few minutes. During this time of hot flashes, you may experience dizziness, insomnia, headaches, fatigue, etc. The best way to deal with these symptoms is to indulge in activities that help in relaxing the mind and body. Again, ask your health practitioner for a recommended list of activities.

Bladder Infection and Stress Incontinence

Bladder infection, commonly caused by diseases like urethritis and cystitis, is another postmenopause symptom. Infection in the bladder or urethra can cause you to experience a burning sensation while urinating, along with lower back pain. Due to this you may develop stress incontinence where you lose the ability to control the passage of urine and it is said to leak out while doing certain activities like laughing, sneezing, running, coughing, lifting, etc.

Bone Pain and Fractures

Postmenopause bones are likely to become weak, leading to low bone density. Due to this, you may be at a high risk of developing osteoporosis and bone pain. This also increases the chance that you may experience bone fractures and leg cramps during this period of your life.

How Long Does Menopausal Symptoms Last?

The answer to this question will not be the same for all women, however, for some it may last only for two to three months. I have also known women that dealt with these symptoms anywhere between two and ten years. As these symptoms usually cause discomfort and can also be an indicator of a serious problem, consulting your health practitioner will help in relieving the symptoms as well as curing the underlying problem.

Treatment for Postmenopausal Symptoms

Some postmenopausal symptoms require specific treatment according to the cause, but most of them can be cured with the help of natural remedies. If the symptoms are caused due to hormonal imbalance, your health practitioner may recommend hormone replacement therapy. Your doctor can conduct several tests to see if there are any problems in the reproductive system. If so, a course of treatment will then be recommended. Exercising regularly and following a balanced diet also are important to remaining fit and fighting diseases that can occur during postmenopause. One may also require multivitamin and mineral supplements as suggested earlier to get rid of some of the postmenopausal symptoms.

As a preventive measure, it is important for you to undergo regular checkups and tests like pelvic exams, mammograms, pap smears, etc. to prevent any kind of health problems associated with the postmenopausal stage.

Postmenopause And Self-Esteem

The start of menopause does not have to be a blow to your confidence. It is so important to remember that this life is not a rehearsal, and that you have only one go round this side of heaven. It is imperative that you remain positive and increase your sense of self-worth during this transitional time in your life.

Postmenopause is a time of transition or change and, as with any significant change in your life (i.e. puberty, marriage, or parenthood), it may be accompanied by feelings of increased vulnerability or even insecurity. As you enter this stage, you will be confronted with a number of issues that can affect the way you see and feel about yourself. These issues often include physical symptoms such as weight gain, hair loss, or dry skin, as well as psychological confusion about how to navigate the transition from one stage of life to another. Emotionally, it can also be tough to deal with the negative stereotypes and attitudes that society traditionally has about aging. Fortunately, times are changing. The view that menopause is the beginning of the end is outdated and untrue. In many ways, it's actually the beginning of an exciting and dynamic period in your life.

Postmenopause Self-Esteem And Success Stories

If you are feeling apprehensive about what postmenopause will bring, it may help to note how other women have successfully navigated its emotional ups and downs. In fact, many women find postmenopause actually ushers in a new way of thinking about their life, one in which confidence, self-acceptance, and self-awareness can be more deeply felt and easily expressed.

Lisa, a lovely lady of fifty-seven years, came in to speak with me about her retirement and life thereafter. We spoke for some time, then I suggested a couple of career paths that fit her temperament. She became so excited about one particular path—personal coaching and public speaking. She asked how to get started. I made a few suggestions and she asked if I would coach her. I enthusiastically said, "Yes!" The rest was history. When talking about the positive boost that postmenopause has brought to her self-esteem, she says, "I feel more confident, as if I can throw away all the nonsense in life and focus more clearly on the things that matter most to me."

Lisa's feelings reflect the findings of a study done by Elavsky S, McAluley E. at Pennsylvania State University. That study examined how postmenopausal women experienced growing older and becoming middle-aged. A majority of the study's participants said that over the course of menopause, they had become more competent and gained a greater sense of freedom. They also reported that they had cultivated a better understanding of possibilities of personal development, which in the end enabled them to hold on to their own opinions and better speak their mind.

Society and Menopause

In the 1980s, one of my colleagues was dismissed from his job for including in an evaluation of one of the clerks the phrase: "Her attitude was always like she is going through menopause." The clerk complained to the union and my colleague was fired for using offensive language. I don't know if the clerk was going through menopause or not, but until recently men would say that about women who spoke up for themselves. Women who were going through menopause felt they were cursed to a life of solitude and asexuality. You may remember your mother or grandmother refusing to talk about menopause—she may not even have acknowledged that she was going through it. This was because society looked down on menopause as unnatural. No books or pamphlets were available to read then, and if you so much as snapped at someone, it was evidence that you were definitely going through "the change." Today, we are witnessing a huge change in the perception of menopause. In part, this is due to that fact that women live over a third of their lives after menopause, in a period called postmenopause. Also, larger numbers of women are now entering menopause earlier thanks to the baby boomer generation. Women who are postmenopausal no longer have to be an old spinster. Postmenopausal women can be business people, homemakers, writers, travelers, pastors, and lovers. If you are postmenopausal, you now have the freedom to enjoy your life without having to hide your body or your emotional self. Society no longer views menopause as a sign of asexuality, but instead as a natural part of womanhood.

Well-Being After Menopause

If you are going through menopause or perimenopause, you may still be worried about how your life is going to be after it's all over. You are probably a little scared about how your body will feel, how your mood will be, and whether or not you will be able to enjoy life in the same way. Well, put your fears to rest, because life after menopause can be quite enjoyable.

Hormone Replacement Therapy

Replacement therapy can become a double-edged sword for your self-esteem. At menopause, most women are confronted with the decision of whether to begin prescription *hormone replacement therapy* (HRT) or not. It is not always an easy choice. While HRT can help ease or even eliminate uncomfortable or problematic menopausal symptoms, it can also be a source of certain serious medical issues. In addition, as a menopause therapy, it will probably be useful only for a few years, since HRT is now generally recommended only for short-term use. If you choose HRT, the prescribed hormones can sometimes help to maintain or improve your self-esteem by easing symptoms. Your physical changes may or may not slow down, concentration issues may improve, and your sex drive may return to premenopausal levels. On the flip side, if you take HRT but do not feel very comfortable with your choice, you may find your self-esteem suffering, especially if your peers are foregoing the hormones or have strong views against using hormone therapy. In any case, it is critical to think through not only your medical options for treating your particular menopausal symptoms, but also how you can best cope with your psychological needs. Then you need to discuss any treatment plan carefully with your physician/health practitioner. This will help you develop a well-rounded plan that will fit both your health needs and your life circumstances.

Tips For Maintaining A Positive Self-Image During Postmenopause

To navigate menopause successfully, you will have to use your transitional and transformative time to come to an acceptance of the changes that postmenopause brings and to develop a renewed sense of self. With the right approach, postmenopause can bring you greater confidence and a sense of empowerment to your life.

Recommendations for Boosting Your Self-Esteem:

- **Exercise!** Exercise not only helps you to offset the slight weight gain that may accompany menopause, but also offers your self-esteem a natural boost. One study showed that menopausal women who walked or did yoga regularly felt better both physically and emotionally and were more confident in their abilities.
- **Maintain a healthy diet.** Eating correctly will do more than help keep off that extra weight that can result from a slower metabolism, but good nutrition can also help address a range of other symptoms associated with postmenopause, including anxiety, mood swings, and insomnia. Make sure your diet has plenty of whole grains, fruits, vegetables, legumes, probiotics,

and almond milk. (It has 50% more calcium than dairy milk.) Use these products so you can be as healthy and fit as you possibly can.

- **Embrace the positive.** "For as he thinketh in his heart, so *is* he . . ." (Prov. 23:7). Think about expanding your horizons. *"A person is limited only by the thoughts that he chooses." James Allen* Life should be about more than just simply surviving menopause. In fact, many women report discovering greater freedom and increased self-confidence as they pass through menopause. So concentrate on embracing these changes while rediscovering the positive aspects of your life, and use the time to begin sampling new things and exploring different possibilities. Creating positive outlets in your life will continue to enhance your self-esteem and give you a greater sense of purpose.

- **Empower yourself.** Gone are the days when women had to suffer in silence through menopause. Today, many resources are available to help you chart your own course. So read up, get educated, and then discuss your ideas or concerns with your health practitioner and other women going through the same process. Research suggests that women who are more informed about the choices they have and the challenges that postmenopause may bring, are that much more likely to feel positive about the experience.

Emotional Well-Being

A study by Debbie Paddington Diopn stated that 75% of women reported they were having more fun in their everyday lives, and 93% reported an increase in their independence during menopause. Menopause can be a time when new doors open up for you. You may find yourself having the freedom to explore new job options, travel, or enjoy leisure activities. Many women also find that they have time for greater self-exploration.

Some women will find that their mood may lower at certain times after menopause. Increased financial responsibilities, health concerns, and work problems can all contribute to low mood. Pile this on top of the physical changes that you have undergone, and it just may be too much. If you find yourself very unhappy, speak with your doctor, as treatments are available. You may also want to look into joining a menopause support group.

Sexual Well-Being And The Postmenopausal Woman

The country and western song that declares "older women are beautiful lovers" finds support in a new study showing sexual satisfaction in women increases with age. After menopause, you may find yourself experiencing greater levels of satisfaction than you did at any other time in your life. As mentioned before in a recent study by Rick Nauert Ph.D., many postmenopausal women wonder what their sex life will be like once they are going through or have completed menopause. Some worry that they will lose their libido or that their partner will no longer be interested in them sexually. A recent study in the UK found that most postmenopausal women actually have a better sex life than they did before menopause. Sixty-five percent reported being happier in their sex lives and this may be due to the lack of concern over unplanned pregnancies. As a postmenopausal woman, you may find yourself free to enjoy sex now that many of your worries associated with sex no longer apply. You may also have an easier time reaching orgasm, and be more likely to experience multiple orgasms during intercourse.

It is true that a small percentage of women do experience a reduced sex drive during and after menopause. Quite often this is due to physical changes in your body, such as vaginal dryness, which can make sex uncomfortable. Emotional concerns can also impact your sex drive after menopause. If you are worried about the way your body looks or the way your partner may react to your body, this could impact your sex drive negatively. Health concerns such as heart disease or osteoporosis as may also affect your desire to have sex. If a lowered sex drive is becoming a problem for you or your partner, discuss it with your health care practitioner, this is not difficult to treat.

What Are Some Causes of Low Libido in Women?

The word *libido* not only refers to the desire for sex, but also sexual thoughts, fantasies, responsiveness and willingness to engage in sexual activity. When decreased libido causes personal distress, the term *hypoactive sexual desire disorder* (HSDD) is used. Keep in mind, however, that "normal" sexual desire and activity may be very different for different people, from multiple times a week to several times a month. There is no simple on-off switch for a woman's sexual desire. There are a multitude of internal and external factors that influence sexual feelings. Variables that influence libido include medical conditions, medications, relationship issues, depression, body image, hormone levels, personal and job stress, and living situations. Sexual desire is also strongly related to underlying good health. Women with chronic health conditions are more likely to report decreased sexual activity and low libido.

At What Age Does Low Libido Occur?

Decreased desire can occur at any age, but in younger women hormone levels are generally high and less likely to be a factor. Fear of pregnancy or disease, feelings of guilt about sexual activity due to cultural or religious beliefs, a traumatic sexual experience, or self-consciousness about appearance may contribute to low libido. Medications such as birth control pills, antidepressants, blood pressure pills, or drugs to treat or prevent cancer can adversely affect libido in women at any age. Postmenopausal women are more likely to experience hot flashes, dryness, or discomfort with intercourse, which often affects desire. Keep in mind that even in the absence of a specific problem, sexual desire decreases somewhat as we age.

How Do You Treat Low Libido?

A "one size fits all" approach doesn't work. If medications for health conditions are contributing to low libido, there are often alternative choices. For postmenopausal and even some premenopausal clients, hormone therapy with estrogen, progestin, or testosterone may be appropriate. Lifestyle modifications including a balanced diet, maintaining a healthy weight, and even fifteen minutes of exercise a day can improve self-image and boost sexual energy. Setting aside special time for sexual activity can heighten pleasure and satisfaction: romantic lighting, music, or lingerie can set the stage. Long-term relationships can suffer from the same routine and the same moves. Surprise your partner or ask your mate to surprise you. Explore each other's fantasies and try some of them out, even if those fantasies include sex toys. Making a conscious effort to think about sex once or twice a day can be of great help. Our brain is a potent aphrodisiac.

There are no herbal supplements that are scientifically endorsed by the U.S. Food and Drug Administration as being medically effective for treating low sex drive in women, according to the Discovery Channel. However, many cultures and medical professionals have used herbal supplements to help women regain that spark in the bedroom. The supplements can work in a variety of ways, from helping promote a sense of well-being to stimulating the sensitivity of the clitoris. Both women and men report that the maca plant can stimulate the libido and sexual function by regulating hormone levels in the body, according to Discovery Health. It also notes that the modern use of maca as a way to boost sexual function is on the rise. Other herbs that have shown to be a sexual stimulant in women are damiana leaf, l-arginine plus, and kava. Before using any herbal supplements, please see a competent physician.

What Role Does Stress and Other Mental Health Issues Play in Low Libido?

Women today have many things competing for their time and energy. Approximately three-quarters of a woman's time is consumed by their job, family, food-shopping, meal preparation, managing the household, homework, and after-school activities. Even with a mate who shares some of the responsibilities, it can feel overwhelming. By the time there is a pause in your hectic day, sleep may become your body's first priority. Additional stress in the relationship between you and your mate can push libido to the back burner. A good question to ask yourself is, *"Is your libido on vacation?"* In a survey conducted by the Hypoactive Sexual Desire Disorder Registry published in 2010, about 60% of women cited stress or fatigue as contributing factors to their low sex drive, more than 40% described dissatisfaction with their appearance, 20 to 25% described dissatisfaction with their mate's technique, and 20% described dissatisfaction with the relationship. In postmenopausal women, 67% reported menopausal symptoms as causing low desire. Try to identify your reason for your low libido however, whatever you decide to do, please do not suffer in silence.

What Other Menopausal Problems May Adversely Affect Your Sexual Life?

It is fair to say that many women have a great time in bed after they pass menopause; others do not. These are some problems that can occur:

- **Night sweats and hot flashes**. This can be counterproductive to relaxation and romance. At night, such symptoms produce an intolerable feeling of heat, often accompanied by profuse sweating, and even a feeling of acute claustrophobia. If the sufferer has to throw off the bed sheets and open the windows when night sweats are at their worst, she's not going to feel like absorbing even more body heat from her sexual mate.
- **Estrogen deficiency** can bring about vaginal dryness and thinning of the vaginal lining. The lack of lubrication and support for the vaginal walls can reduce arousal during sex and increase friction, which in turn may produce soreness, burning, or irritation.
- **Irregular periods** can make the timing of spontaneous love-making difficult. (Menopause shouldn't really cause irregular periods; if this is the case, consult your doctor.)
- **Stress urinary incontinence (SUI)** can occasionally arise during love-making—or during a climax.

- **Physical Symptoms** such as dry skin, changes in the shape of their breasts, and a gradual redistribution of weight away from their breasts towards their waistline.
- **Loss of libido** can occur. Minorities of women complain that after menopause they simply lose their desire for sex. Husbands may feel rejected because of this, and so relationship difficulties can arise, or even extra-marital affairs.
- **Psychological symptoms** such as mood swings, insomnia, and depression can make it difficult to enjoy sex.

The good news is that all these problems can usually be remedied—chiefly through common sense advice from a competent physician (or from a therapist who is experienced in dealing with menopause problems), together with sympathy, understanding, and love from our mate. There are also many natural therapies and treatments that can boost your libido.

An Important Note about Family Planning

A woman's fertility starts to fall after about the age of thirty-five, but many women have been surprised when they have become pregnant unexpectedly in their late forties or even early fifties. Late pregnancy can and does happen, so it is important to think about contraception—even after the menopause.

The recommended advice is:

- If you start menopause at fifty or over, you should use contraception for twelve months after your last period.
- If you are under fifty when you start menopause you should continue to use contraception for two years after your last period.
- If you started taking HRT (*Hormone replacement therapy*) before your last period, you should continue using contraception until the age of fifty-three to be on the safe side. Please remember that HRT is not a contraceptive.

The truth is that there is no reason why you cannot continue to enjoy a happy and satisfying sex life during and after menopause, if you choose to. In counseling with women of menopausal age and talking with colleagues, I have found that many women enjoy wonderful sex lives after they have passed menopause and continue to do so for a very long time. We have even uncovered some evidence that:

- Women who are interested in sex are more likely to be orgasmic after their change of life than younger females.
- Women are also more likely to be more multi-orgasmic after menopause.

There are three main reasons for this:

1. After the change of life most women are glad to be worry-free about contraception.
2. By the time you are approximately 50 years of age, you should have gained a great deal of love-making knowledge, experience and skill to make it an enjoyable experience for you and your mate.
3. By this time, you should have a mate who actually knows what he is doing in bed. Of course, a few postmenopausal women—notably certain celebrities—decide to take "boy toys" as lovers.

Case in Point

A few years ago a couple came in for premarital counseling— she was fifty-three and he was twenty-two., He was so young I smelled the Similac on his breath. She was infatuated with his youth and stamina. Two months later she called saying he found a younger girl friend and left her. She said she would never again trust another man. I later ran into her at a local social and she introduced a lady to me as her new roommate. The next day she called my office and asked what I thought of her roommate. After I told her that she seemed to be a nice lady, she informed me that the "roommate" was her lover and that I should not think badly of her because everybody needs love. I put her at ease by letting her know that I could not judge her. Later that week, she visited my office and we talked about the guilt she felt in her new relationship. She expressed that she was not really happy in the relationship because she was not a lesbian and did not mean for it to happen. Her roommate was actually looking for intimacy but was confusing sex with intimacy. She said that she would rather be in a relationship with a man but men in her age group lack the patience to bring her to the place of sexual satisfaction.

Men and women in their forties usually crave sex more than at any other time in their adult life, according to several studies. However, because women in this age group quite often have a pelvic floor that weakens where the vagina starts losing its elasticity; they do not easily get aroused. Consequently, men of this age do not spend the needed time it may take to bring their women to climax before he does. This may be due to selfishness and haste. A younger man has the patience, sexual energy, and stamina to be there at the time she exhales.

Again keep in mind that your estrogen levels start declining at this age so you might experience hot flashes or sudden feelings of warmth, flushing, sweating, chills, and feelings of disorientation or confusion. Hot flashes last five to 10 minutes and may cause sleep disturbances due to the soaking sweats that occur with them. Also, dopamine is known to play an essential role in the sex life. Once you are in a predictable and stable relationship, the dopamine in the brain quiets down. Doing exciting and new things with your mate can again kick start the production of dopamine in your body.

Do not neglect sex just because you are in your forties or fifties. The more sex you have, the closer you will feel to your mate. Your partner will also be more romantically inclined towards you and this will generally increase the intimacy level for both of you. For a healthy relationship, frequent sex is essential and reaching your forties is no reason why you should not have sex frequently. Try different things, see what works for you and keep going at it.

Living a Balanced Life

The key to living your life to the fullest is balance. How can you live your life to the fullest if there are areas of your life that are suffering? For example, maybe you are successful in your career, but your family life is not happy. Or maybe you are a very knowledgeable woman but you are battling an illness. To live your life to the fullest, I believe there are five areas of life that needs to be balanced. Those five areas are *spirituality, mind, body, relationship*, and *work*. Here are the details:

1. **Spirituality**
   This area deals with your conscience, values, and principles. It also deals with your relationship with the Infinite. I call him God. Your spirituality is where your life purpose and meaning come from. In my opinion, the fact that it gives meaning to your life makes it the most important of all five. But it doesn't mean that you should focus only on developing your spirituality. Even if your spirituality is strong, you will not live your life to the fullest if you do not develop the other four areas in balance.

2. **Mind**
   This area deals with your desire to learn. In this fast-changing world, your ability to absorb new skills and knowledge becomes increasingly important In fact, I think this is the most important skill you should master. To have a strong desire to learn, be sure to develop your intellectual hunger.

3. **Body**
   This area deals with your physical health. Since your body is the means through which you conduct your actions, it is important to keep your body in tip-top shape. Not only you should prevent yourself from being sick, you should also

thrive to have the high-level of energy you need to accomplish your tasks with speed and enthusiasm.

4. Relationship

This area deals with your relationships with your family, friends, and colleagues. Relationships are what make your life beautiful. The greatest feeling of fulfillment does not come from your achievements; it comes from your relationships.

What is your most important need in this life? No, it is not money. It's not your achievements or recognition. The most important thing we all need is *love*. We all need to love and to be loved. Unfortunately, sometimes we are so obsessed with other things that we forget how beautiful it is to love and be loved. Do not let this happen to you. Give yourself permission to love others and be loved. Allow yourself to feel how wonderful it is to be loved. Give a taste of your love to someone. We can only do this through relationships. This is the only way. There is no other way you can love and be loved but through relationships.

5. Work

This area deals with your career and achievements. This is the output of your life; your productivity is measured here. If you want to be a productive person, you should increase your output in this area.

These five areas should serve as a framework on which to build your life. There should be strong and balanced growth in all these areas. To grow your life in all of these areas, you should allocate your daily time and energy around them. You should designate a block of time for each: spirituality, mind, body, relationship, and work. Whenever you feel that one area is under developed, you should put more effort in that area.

Moving Forward from Here

At any stage of your life, you can move forward. What is stopping you from fulfilling your purpose and achieving your dreams? Like thousand of women you may find yourself repeatedly stuck in the same old rut—relationships, finances, career, health, or spiritual life. Maybe you want to start exercising, find a better job, get out of debt, launch a business, deepen your friendships, practice a new spiritual discipline or pursue some other goal. The question is, *"What's Really Holding You Back?"*

What Should I Give Up?

1. **Letting the opinions of others control your life.** People know your name, not your story. They have heard what you have done, but not what you have been through. So take their opinions of you with a grain of salt. In the end, it is not what others think, it's what you think about yourself that counts. Sometimes you have to do exactly what is best for you and your life, not what is best for everyone else.

2. **The shame of past failures.** You will fail sometimes, and that's okay. The faster you accept this, the faster you can get on with being brilliant. Your past does not equal your future. Just because you failed yesterday, or today, or even a moment ago, doesn't have any impact on the current moment. All that matters is what you do right now.

3. **Being indecisive about what you want.** You will never leave where you are until you decide where you would rather be. It's all about finding and pursuing your passion. Neglecting passion blocks creative flow. When you're passionate, you are energized. Likewise, when you lack passion, your energy is low and unproductive. Energy is everything when it comes to being successful. Make a decision to figure out what you want, and then pursue it passionately.

4. **Procrastinating on the goals that matter to you.** There are two primary choices in life: to accept conditions as they exist, or accept the responsibility for changing them. Follow your intuition. Do not give up trying to do what you really want to do. When there is love and inspiration, you can't go wrong. And whatever it is you want to do, do it now. There are only so many tomorrows. Trust me, in a year from now, you will wish you had started today.

5. **Choosing to do nothing.** You do not get to choose how you are going to die, or when. You can only decide how you are going to live, right now. Every day is a new chance to choose. Choose to change your perspective. Choose to flip the switch in your mind from negative to positive. Choose to turn on the light and stop fretting about with insecurity and doubt. Choose to do work that you are proud of. Choose to see the best in others, and to show your best to others. Choose to truly LIVE, right now, today.

6. **Your need to be right.** If you keep on saying you're right, even if you are right now, eventually you will be wrong. Aim for success, but never give up your right to be wrong. Because when you do, you will also lose your ability to learn new things and move forward with your life.

7. **Running from problems that should be fixed.** We make life harder than it has to be. The difficulties started when conversations became texting, feelings became subliminal, sex became a game, the word "love" fell out of context, trust faded as honesty waned, insecurities became a way of living, jealously became a habit, being hurt started to feel natural, and running away from it all became our solution. Stop running! Face these issues, fix the problems, communicate, appreciate, show gratitude, forgive, and LOVE the people in your life who deserve it.

8. **Making excuses rather than decisions.** Life is a continuous exercise in creative problem solving. A mistake doesn't become

a failure until you refuse to correct it. Thus, most long-term failures are the outcome of people who make excuses instead of decisions.

9. **Overlooking the positive points in your life.** What you see often depends entirely on what you are looking for. Do your best and surrender the rest. When you stay stuck in regret of the life you think you should have had, you end up missing the beauty of what you do have. You will have a hard time ever being happy if you are not thankful for the good things in your life right now.

10. **Not appreciating the present moment.** We do not remember days, we remember moments. Too often we try to accomplish something big without realizing that the greatest part of life is made up of the little things. Live authentically and cherish each precious moment of your journey. Because when you finally arrive at your desired destination, I guarantee you, another journey will begin. So, *"What's Really Holding You Back?"*

Chapter Eight

ALONG THE WAY YOU MAY EXPERIENCE—DEPRESSION ITS CAUSES, SYMPTOMS, AND TREATMENT

Initially, I was not going to make this chapter a part of this book. However, after viewing an episode of the Dr. Oz TV show about depression among women, I was alarmed at the national statistics given by his panel of mental health professionals. Their findings verified what I assumed from my own encounters while counseling and listening to women or at my conferences and workshops. Though I assumed their findings to be correct; it was still alarming. The fact is that everyone occasionally feels blue or sad, but these feelings are usually fleeting and pass within a couple of days. On the other hand, when a woman has a depressive disorder, it interferes with her daily life and normal functioning, and causes pain for both the one with the disorder and those who care about her. In fact, according to the National Mental Health Association, about one in every eight women will develop depression at some point during her lifetime. Depression is a serious condition that can affect a person's social life, relationships, career, self-worth, and purpose. Depression affects both men and women alike, but each year more women are likely to be diagnosed than men. Efforts to explain this are ongoing as researchers are exploring certain factors—biological, social, etc. that are associated with the disease. These factors are, however, unique to each person.

The Best Way of Understanding Depression

If you're constantly feeling sad, guilty, tired, and just generally "down in the dumps," you may be suffering from major depression. But the good news is that depression is treatable, and the more you understand about depression's particular implications for and impact on women, the more equipped you will be to tackle the condition head on.

Though debilitating and serious, most women with depression never seek treatment, although with treatment the majority of women, (even those with the most severe depression), can get better.

Are There Different Forms of Depression?

There are several forms of depressive disorders that occur in both women and men. The most common are major depressive disorder and dysthymic disorder. Minor depression is also a form.

Major depressive disorders are characterized by a combination of symptoms that interfere with the person's ability to work, sleep, study, eat, and enjoy once-pleasurable activities. Major depression is disabling and prevents the person from functioning normally. Some women will experience an episode of major depression only once in their lifetime, but it also can reoccur throughout her life.

Dysthymic disorder is characterized by depressive symptoms that are long-term (e.g., two years or longer) but less severe than those of major depression. Dysthymia may not disable you, but it could prevent you from functioning normally or feeling well. Women with dysthymia may also experience one or more episodes of major depression during their lifetime.

Depression comes in several varieties; some forms of this disorder have slightly different characteristics and may develop under different and unique circumstances. However, not all psychologists or other mental health professionals agree on how to characterize and define these forms of depression. Let us take a look at the following:

- **Psychotic depression** occurs when a severe depressive illness is accompanied by some form of psychosis, such as a break with reality. A woman may see, hear, smell, or feel things that others can't detect (hallucinations or having strong beliefs that are false (delusions) such as believing she is the first lady of United States of America or the pastor's wife when she is not.
- **Seasonal affective disorder** (SAD) is characterized by a depressive illness during the winter months, when there is less natural sunlight. The depression generally lifts during spring and summer. SAD may be effectively treated with light therapy, but nearly half of those with SAD do not respond to light therapy alone. Antidepressant medication and psychotherapy also can reduce SAD symptoms, either alone or in combination with light therapy.
- **Bipolar disorder, also called manic-depressive illness**, may not be as common as major depression or dysthymia; however, it is becoming the pillar of the most undiagnosed depressive disorder in our country today. Bipolar disorder is characterized by cycling mood changes: from extreme highs (e.g., mania) to extreme lows (e.g., depression).

A Few Basic Signs of Depression

Some women describe depression as "living in a black hole" or having a feeling of impending doom. However, some depressed people don't feel sad at all—they may feel lifeless, empty, and apathetic, even feel angry, aggressive, and restless.

Whatever the symptoms, depression is different from normal sadness in that it engulfs your day-to-day life. As stated previously, it interferes with your ability to work, study, eat, sleep, and have fun. The feelings of helplessness, hopelessness, and worthlessness are intense and unrelenting, with little, if any, relief.

The symptoms of depression in women are somewhat different from that found in men. Women with depressive illnesses do not all experience the same symptoms. In addition, the severity and frequency of symptoms, and how long they last, will vary depending on the individual and her particular illness. Signs and symptoms of depression in women include but are not limited to:

- Persistent sad, anxious or "empty" feelings
- Feelings of hopelessness and/or pessimism
- Irritability, restlessness, anxiety
- Feelings of guilt, worthlessness and/or helplessness
- Loss of interest in activities or hobbies once pleasurable, including sex
- Fatigue and decreased energy
- Difficulty concentrating, remembering details and making decisions
- Insomnia, waking up during the night, or excessive sleeping
- Overeating, or appetite loss
- Thoughts of suicide, suicide attempts
- Persistent aches or pains, headaches, cramps, or digestive problems that do not ease even with treatment.

The Causes of Depression Vary

Scientists are still examining many potential causes for and contributing factors to women's increased risk for depression. It is likely that genetic, biological, chemical, hormonal, environmental, psychological, and social factors all intersect to contribute to depression.

Genetic Depression

"If a woman has a family history of depression, she may be more at risk of developing the illness. However, this is not a hard and fast rule. Depression can occur at any time with or without a family history of depression; and women from families with a history of depression may not develop depression themselves. Genetics research indicates that the risk for developing depression likely involves the combination of multiple genes with environmental or other factors." *Nature Reviews Genetics* Vol. 9, 527-540 (July 2008)

Chemical and Hormone Depression

Brain chemistry appears to be a significant factor in depressive disorders. While working at The New York State Office of Mental Health, I had the opportunity to view many brain scans of people suffering from depression. They all looked different from those of people without depression. The parts of the brain responsible for regulating mood, thinking, sleep, appetite and behavior appear to be different in patterns. Scientists are also studying the influence of female hormones, which changes throughout life. Researchers have shown that hormones directly affect the brain chemistry that controls emotions and mood. Specific times during a woman's life are of particular interest, including puberty; the times before menstrual periods; before, during, and just after pregnancy (postpartum); and just prior to and during menopause (perimenopause).

Premenstrual Dysphoric Disorder

"Some women may be susceptible to a severe form of premenstrual syndrome called Premenstrual Dysphoric Disorder (PMDD). Women affected by PMDD typically experience depression, anxiety, irritability and mood swings the week before menstruation, in such a way that interferes with their normal functioning. Women with debilitating PMDD do not necessarily have unusual hormone changes, but they do have different responses to these changes." *Mary M. Gallenberg, M.D of The Mayo Clinic*

Postpartum Depression

Women are particularly vulnerable to depression after giving birth, when hormonal and physical changes and the new responsibility of caring for a newborn can be overwhelming. Many new mothers experience a brief episode of mild mood changes known as the "baby blues;" but some will suffer from postpartum depression, a much more serious condition that requires active treatment and emotional support for the new mother. One study found that postpartum women are at an increased risk for several mental disorders—including depression—for several months after childbirth.

Menopause

Hormonal changes increase during the transition between premenopause and menopause. While some women may transition into menopause without any problems with mood, others experience an increased risk for depression. This seems to occur even among women without a history of depression. Depression becomes less common for women during the postmenopause period.

Stress

Stressful life events such as trauma, loss of a loved one, difficulty in relationship or any stressful situation—whether welcomed or unwelcomed—often occurs before a depressive episode. Additional work and home responsibilities, caring for children and aging parents, abuse, and poverty may also trigger a depressive episode. Evidence suggests that women respond differently than men to these events, making them more prone to depression. In fact, research indicates that when women respond in such a way that prolongs their feelings of stress, there is an increased risk for depression. It is unclear, however, why some women faced with enormous challenges develop depression, and some with similar challenges do not.

The Link Between Intimate Partner Violence And Depression

Women who have experienced violence from their partner (intimate partner violence) are at a higher risk of becoming depressed. They may also be at an increased risk of experiencing intimate partner violence, according to a study by International Researchers published in *PLOS Medicine*.

In her study, Ms. Karen Devries of the London School of Hygiene & Tropical Medicine, found that women who have been abused by a partner are more likely to be depressed and depressed women are more likely to be abused by a partner. Furthermore, this cycle of partner violence and depression seems to only be true for women, while men are seemingly unaffected.

Though I have not done the kind of study Ms. Devries has, I have spoken to enough women in domestic violent relationships to conclude that the vast majority of these women are also suffering from depression and a loss of self-esteem. Their intimate partners in these relationships are quite aware of this and use it to their advantage against the abused and depressed partner. There are other researchers who discovered women were twice as likely to develop depression if they had been physically abused by a partner in the past. On the flip side, women with depression have double the odds of experiencing partner abuse in her future.

Depression and Other Coexisting Illnesses

Often there are several other illnesses that coexist with depression—i.e. eating disorders such as anorexia nervosa, bulimia nervosa and others, especially among women. Anxiety disorders, such as post-traumatic stress disorder (PTSD), obsessive-compulsive disorder, panic disorder, social phobia and generalized anxiety disorder, also sometimes accompany depression. Women are more prone than men to having a co-existing anxiety disorder. Women suffering from PTSD, which can result after she has endured a terrifying ordeal, such as abandonment, domestic abuse, or rape and sexual abuse are especially prone to suffer from depression.

How Does Depression Affect Adolescent Girls?

Richard McKeon, Chief of the Suicide Prevention Branch at the U.S. Substance Abuse and Mental Health Services Administration, reported in April 2013 that girls are experiencing major depressive episodes around the time of puberty. This is earlier than in years past, and really points to the need for early interventions in the form of treatments. The report, based on a large national survey conducted annually to assess drug use and mental health, found that girls aged 12 to 17 were at triple the risk of experiencing a major depressive episode when compared to boys (12% vs. 4.5%). It's unclear why these gender disparities exist, but they're probably due to multiple factors including biological vulnerability and, perhaps, the higher rates of sexual abuse among girls.

Prior to adolescence, both girls and boys experience depression at the same rate; however, at adolescence girls become more likely to experience episode depression than boys. There are several possible reasons for this imbalance. Chief among the reasons are that the biological and hormonal changes that occur during puberty likely contribute to the sharp increase in rates of depression among adolescent girls. In addition, research has suggested that girls are more likely than boys to continue feeling bad after experiencing difficult situations or events, suggesting they are more prone to depression. With all the progress we seem to have made in equality between boy and girls, I have found that girls tend to doubt themselves and their abilities to solve problems and view their problems as unsolvable more so than boys. There is also the public demand on body image. Girls with concerns of how they look and how others view them are more likely to be preoccupied with not measuring up to the image in their head. If this preoccupation continues, they will be more likely to have depressive symptoms as well.

How Does Depression Affect Older Women?

As with the adolescence girls, more adult women than men experience depression, but rates decrease among women after menopause. Evidence suggests that depression in postmenopausal women generally occurs in women with prior histories of depression. In any case, depression is not a normal part of aging.

There are several other causes of emotional debilitation among both sexes such as: the death of a spouse or loved one, moving from work into retirement, or dealing with a chronic illness that can leave women and men alike feeling sad or distressed. After a period of adjustment, many older women can regain their emotional balance, but others do not and may develop depression. When older women do suffer from depression, it may be overlooked because older adults may be less willing to discuss feelings of sadness or grief, or they may have less obvious symptoms of depression. As a result, their doctors may be less likely to suspect or spot it.

It is not far-fetched for older adults to experience depression for the first time later in life because of restricted blood flow, a condition called ischemia. Over time, blood vessels become less flexible. They may harden and prevent blood from flowing normally to the body's organs, including the brain. If this occurs, an older adult with no family or personal history of depression may develop what some doctors call "vascular depression."

In many cases, depression, even the most severe cases, is a highly treatable disorder. As with many illnesses, the earlier the treatment can begin, the more effective it is and the greater the likelihood that a recurrence of the depression can be prevented. The first step to getting appropriate treatment is to visit a competent physician. Elderly adults can become depressed because of the number of medications that they are taking. Keep an eye out for certain viruses or thyroid disorders these can also be the cause of many depressive symptoms. A physician can rule out these possibilities by conducting a physical examination, interview, and/or lab tests, depending on the medical condition. Some older adults become depressed because of loneliness; most of their friends have made their transition to another life, leaving them alone without the mobility to get around as they once did.

Treatments

A person with depression can be treated a number of different ways once they are diagnosed. The most common treatment methods are medication and psychotherapy. I have also found that prayer, love, involvement, and visitation from other people can help to keep a depressed individual from isolation. Keep in mind that these are not substitutes for medication or psychotherapy.

Prescribed Medication

Most anti-depressants work to normalize naturally occurring brain chemicals called neurotransmitters, notably serotonin and norepinephrine. Other antidepressants work on the neurotransmitter, dopamine. Studies of people with depression have found that these particular chemicals are involved in regulating mood, but they are unsure of the exact ways in which they work. The newest and most popular types of antidepressant medications are called selective serotonin reuptake inhibitors (SSRIs) and include:

- fluoxetine (Prozac)
- citalopram(Celexa)
- sertraline (Zoloft)
- paroxetine (Paxil)
- escitalopram (Lexapro)
- fluvoxamine (Luvox)

Serotonin and norepinephrine reuptake inhibitors (SNRI) are similar to the above SSRIs and include:

- venlafaxine (Effexor)
- duloxetine (Cymbalta)

Most antidepressant medications are very toxic and therefore have many side effects. SSRI and SNRI tend to have fewer side effects and are more popular than the older classes of antidepressants, such as tricyclics—named for their chemical structure—and monoamine oxidase inhibitors (MAOIs). However, medications affect everyone differently. There is no one-size-fits-all approach to medication. Therefore, for some people, tricyclics or MAOIs may or may not be the best choice.

The problem with most people taking antidepressants is that they are not told by their physicians of the serious implications when they do not adhere to a restricted diet. People taking MAOI's must adhere to significant food and medicinal restrictions to avoid potentially serious interactions. They must avoid certain foods that contain high levels of the chemical tyramine, which is found in many cheeses, wines and pickles, and some medications including decongestants. Most MAOI's interact with tyramine in such a way that may cause a sharp increase in blood pressure, which may lead to a stroke. Their physicians should not only give a person taking an MAOI a complete list of prohibited foods, medicines and substances but, talk to them about these prohibited foods, and other substances.

All anti-depressants must be taken at the prescribed doses for at least three to four weeks, sometimes longer, according to the physician's direction before they are likely to experience a full effect. They should continue taking the medication for an amount of time specified by their physician, even if they are feeling better, to prevent a relapse of the depression. The decision to stop taking medication should be made by the person and her physician together, and should be done only under the physician's supervision. Some medications need to be gradually weaned to give the body time to adjust. Although they are not habit-forming or addictive, abruptly ending an antidepressant can cause withdrawal symptoms or lead to a relapse. Some individuals, such as those with chronic or recurrent depression, may need to stay on the medication indefinitely.

In addition, if for some reason the first or second medication does not work, be open to trying another. Research funded by NIMH has shown that those who did not get well after taking a first medication often fared better after they switched to a different medication or added another medication, such as a stimulants or anti-anxiety medications. I am not one to suggest taking any medication over natural alternatives to medications, however; in this case I believe it might be the best choice because of the severity of the debilitating ailment. Please realize that neither anti-anxiety medications nor stimulants are effective against depression when taken alone, and both should be taken only under a doctor's close supervision.

Is It Safe To Take Anti-Depressant Medication During Pregnancy?

Not too long ago, it was assumed by doctors that pregnancy was accompanied by a natural feeling of well-being, and that depression during pregnancy rarely if ever occurs. Recent studies, however, have shown that women can have depression while pregnant, especially if they have a prior history of this illness. In fact, the majority of women with a history of depression will likely relapse during pregnancy if they stop taking their antidepressant medication either prior to conception or early in the pregnancy, putting both mother and baby at risk.

In 2004, the U.S. Food and Drug Administration (FDA) issued a warning against the use of SSRI in the late third trimester of pregnancy, suggesting that physicians gradually taper expectant mothers off SSRI in the third trimester to avoid any ill effects on the baby.

It is advisable for expecting mothers to avoid taking their antidepressant medications without first discussing the possibility of doing so with their physician. Keep in mind that these medications do pass across the placental barrier, potentially exposing the developing fetus to the medication. Some research suggests the use of SSRI during pregnancy is associated with miscarriage and/or birth defects, but other studies do not support this. And still other studies have indicated that fetuses exposed to SSRI during the third trimester may be born with "withdrawal" symptoms such as breathing problems, jitteriness, irritability, difficulty feeding, or hypoglycemia. Although some studies suggest that exposure to SSRI in pregnancy may have adverse effects on the infant, generally they are mild and short-lived, and no deaths have been reported. On the flip side, women who stop taking their antidepressant medication during pregnancy increase their risk for developing depression again and may put both themselves and their infant at risk. In light of these mixed results, women and their doctors need to consider the potential risks and benefits to both mother and fetus of taking an anti-depressant during pregnancy, and make decisions based on individual needs and circumstances.

In some cases, a woman and her physician may decide to taper her antidepressant dose during the last month of pregnancy to minimize the newborn's withdrawal symptoms, and after delivery, return to a full dose during the vulnerable postpartum period.

Anti-depressants are excreted in breast milk, usually in very small amounts. The amount an infant receives is usually so small that it does not register in blood tests. Few problems are seen among infants nursing from mothers who are taking antidepressants. However, as with antidepressant use during pregnancy, both the risks and benefits to the mother and infant should be taken into account when deciding whether to take an anti-depressant while breastfeeding.

Anti-Depressant Side Effects

Anti-depressants may cause mild and often temporary but annoying side effects in some people. The most common side effects associated with SSRI and SNRI include:

- Headaches; usually temporary and will subside.
- Nausea; temporary and usually short-lived.
- Insomnia and nervousness (trouble falling asleep or waking often during the night): may occur during the first few weeks but often subside over time or if the dose is reduced.
- Anxiety (e.g., feeling jittery)
- Sexual problems; women can experience sexual problems including reduced sex drive and problems having and enjoying sex

Amarine, MC, Frankenburg, FR, Hensen, J, Reich, DB, and Silk, KR. "Predictions of the 10-year course of borderline personality disorder." American Journal of Psychiatry, 163:827-832, 2006.

It is important to have an understanding of your body; how it feels, acts and responds. Never diagnose yourself or take your feelings light heartedly. If for any reason you feel out of sorts, please speak to your doctor. Do not take your friends' medication and allow them to tell you they had the same thing and this is what they took.

Final Thoughts

I believe that many of you are looking in the wrong direction in your search for self-knowledge and spiritual truth. You have separated the spiritual from everyday living, and thus separated yourselves from experiencing everyday spirituality. The spiritual has become associated with Sunday church services, or the Sabbath, or yoga and meditation, or a trip to Israel, or a tour of a famous European cathedral. I believe praying is a much more spiritual effort than talking about God. We are living secularized lives and yet wondering why life often feels so meaningless and devoid of purpose. The search for real moments and everyday spirituality must begin with a return to and embracing of God. God begins and ends where you already are, right here, and right now. There is nothing else to look for, nothing else to acquire. You already have everything you need to be the woman God created you to be. When He created you he did so because, He had something in mind that only a woman could do.

In order to experience everyday spirituality, you need to remember that you are a spiritual being spending some time in a human body. You are not separate from Spirit; this would be impossible. You are simply spirit disguised in human form. In this way, you are connected to all life. When you separate the spiritual from the everyday, you limit your opportunities for real moments. If you separate the spiritual from the everyday you will miss ordinary miracles and wonders that are put aside for you because you are looking for something flashy, something that screams, "I am special, and I am holy." Don't be so distracted by your search for the extraordinary that you don't recognize the sacred when you encounter it. Real moments of holiness happen when you experience moments of wholeness with yourself, your environment, and the people you encounter in life. As you go through your day, look for holy moments and everyday miracles such as: the hug your child gives you for no reason; a flock of birds flying past a cloud; the beautiful array of fruits and vegetables the earth has produced that are waiting for you at the supermarket; the song playing on the radio that gives you just the message you've been needing to hear; the lone yellow dandelion bursting through the crack in the concrete sidewalk. When you stop and pay attention to holy moments and everyday miracles you will start living with awe and wonder, and participating in a divine love affair with God. You are alive. You are here now. You have another day. That is a blessing. Enjoy the ordinary everyday miracles that make up your life; they will be your most sacred real moments. The purpose of your life is for you to grow into the best human being you can be. Life on earth is a classroom. We are students, here to learn certain lessons. Life is not supposed to just go smoothly. Things are not supposed to be perfect. We are supposed to experience challenges. We are supposed to undergo difficulty. We are here to learn.

"You are a unique, precious, one of a kind treasure of God manifested in the flesh."

Ma'at Hotep

A Word from the Author's Wife

In his latest book, *The Beauty of a Woman*, Dr. Ray Morgan guides us to a healthier way of living and reminds us that turning every issue over to God gives us the strength to make lasting changes. To help us do this, Ray looks deeply into the Four Stages of a Woman as she changes from one to the other, and so many other principles such as:

> Taking responsibility—the choice is ours
> Let go and let God do the heavy lifting
> Learning about our bodies as we journey through
> our Emotional, Physical, and Spiritual stages.

This book is absolutely exceptional. It is so informative with "pure wisdom." I wish I had this book in my younger years. Every woman needs to read and apply the nuggets therein to their lives regardless of her age. It's not too late to take responsibility for our bodies and our souls.

To all my sisters of all ages, I challenge you to open the cover of this phenomenal book and allow your mind to soar emotionally, physically into a beautiful place of beauty. "Draw near to God and He will draw near to you." (James 4:8) Be blessed as you read.

To Dr. Morgan: A beautiful life and a beautiful book.
From my Heart to your Heart,
I love you forever.

Regina Morgan
Associate Director
Insight for the Family, Inc.

A Word from the Author's Daughter

Many people say that a girl's first impression of how she should be treated by a man is through the words and actions of her father. I'm proud to say that I had the best teacher. My father, Dr. Ray Morgan, has impacted my life in many ways. The older I become the more I realize, value and cherish every moment that we continue to share.

I think of how Dad would talk to me when I was a little girl. I never thought of how he was subconsciously building me up emotionally, physically, and spiritually into the woman I am today. I learned to take pride in myself; he taught me morals, values and to be humble and confident all in the same breath. His experience and knowledge in life has made him my #1 go to.

Dad you are my confidante, my hero, and the first love of my life.

I Love You Dad,

Kristal

A Word from the Author's Daughters-in-law

Dr. Morgan offers a timely and holistic approach to the often pondered "Who am I, and what do I need?" at a period when I'm looking introspectively and trying to get to know myself apart from my roles as a wife, mother and educator. "Beauty of a Woman" reveals how the Whole woman is designed, nurtured and made complete at each phase of life, and how her needs change with time, space and experience. Nothing about a woman is simple or compartmentalized. Rather, like a work of art, many colors, textures, and strokes must integrate and change to create a masterpiece! "Beauty of a Woman" is a captivating read that will inform and enthrall male and female audiences alike.

Love you Dad,

V. Thomas M.S., CCC-SLP

When a girl is born, God gives her a father. One who knows her temperament and how to use her temperament as a guide in preparation for what life has to throw at her. While growing up she looks to her father for advice, more specifically about whom to marry. While dating the potential spouse she asks herself, "Is he the one?" The best way to judge is to look at his father.

I am blessed to have a loving, caring, patient husband because of his father. Dr. Morgan (Dad) is the best father-in-law that can be given by God as a guide to help me and other women along our life journey. I am so excited to have this beautiful book "The Beauty of A Woman" to help me to reach the next chapter in my life.

Love,

Hope Morgan

ABOUT THE AUTHOR

Dr. Ray Morgan (Imhotep) and his queen, Regina (Ankhesenamen), are the founders of INSIGHT FOR THE FAMILY, INC., a community-based marriage and family counseling service.

Dr. Ray Morgan is the clinical director of The PER ANKH Clinic of Hope Center for Integrated Health. He has also received extensive training in nutritional, herbal, and homeopathic medicine. He has helped thousands of people to discover the joy of living in divine health.

He has inspired thousands of individuals around the world who have undergone powerful health and emotional transformations in their individual lives by visiting his office and by attending his inspirational health seminars, conferences, and individual counseling sessions.

Dr. Morgan is highly sought after for lectures, conferences and speaking engagements throughout the international community. In his own unique, dynamic and entertaining style, he uplifts and motivates his audiences on a variety of health and emotional topics including detoxifications, health restoration, relationships, personal growth, life coaching, and rites of passage programs. Dr. Morgan retired from The New York State Department of Mental Health. He holds a medical degree and two post-graduate degrees in marriage and family systems. He is a certified member of the American Homeopathic Association; a certified member of the American Association of Christian Counselors; an associate member of the American Society of Christian Therapists; and a clinical member of the International Colonic Therapists.

Dr. Morgan has lectured in Africa, Australia, Belgium, Canada, the Caribbean, Egypt, England, India, New Zealand, and throughout the

United States. His extensive involvement in church and civic affairs has earned him many honors.

Together, Dr. Ray and his Queen, Regina, are blessed to be the parents of four wonderful children: Scott, Kristal, Nekia, Tobias, and three grandchildren: Sakai, Kimari, Sanje, and Adonis.

Ray Morgan, OMD., Ph.D.

Office:
Insight For The Family, Inc.
744 St. Johns Place
Brooklyn, New York 11216
(718) 773-2196

Website:
www.insightforthefamily@yahoo.com

E-mail:
Insightfamily@aol.com

Books:
When Two Become One:
A Diamond in the Making
Published by: Author House Publishing

Food for Thought: 25 Ways to Protect Yourself from
Disease and Promote Excellent Health
Published by: Author House Publishing

Is Money The Problem Or Are You The Problem?
Published by: Insight for the Family, Inc. Publishing

DVDs:
When Two Become One:
A Diamond in the Making
Published by: Insight for the Family, Inc.

Health Emporium
Published by: Insight for the Family, Inc. Publishing

For conferences and workshops, contact:
Insight For The Family, Inc.
744 St. Johns Place
Brooklyn, New York 11216
(718) 773-2196

www.ingramcontent.com/pod-product-compliance
Lightning Source LLC
Chambersburg PA
CBHW030931180526
45163CB00002B/534